The
HERITAGE HERBAL

RECIPES AND REMEDIES FOR MODERN LIVING

SONYA PATEL ELLIS

Foreword by Kim Walker & Vicky Chown
Handmade Apothecary

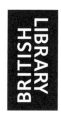

For Sylvester & Iggy

First published in 2020 by
The British Library
96 Euston Road,
London NW1 2DB

Text © Sonya Patel Ellis 2020
Foreword © Kim Walker and Vicky Chown, Handmade Apothecary 2020
Illustrations copyright © 2020 The British Library Board

Cataloguing in Publication Data
A catalogue record for this publication is available from The British Library

ISBN 978 0 7123 5380 9

Design and typesetting by Karin Fremer
Printed and bound by Finidr, Czech Republic

Publisher's Note
The information in this book is strictly informational and for
educational purposes, to inform the reader about traditional remedies
and approaches in herbal medicine. It is not and should not be deemed
to be medical opinion or medical advice, or considered a substitute for the
advice of a medical professional. Moreover, it is not possible to predict every
individual's reactions to a particular remedy, recipe or treatment included in
this book. Please consult a medical professional if you have any health-related
questions, pre-existing conditions, are pregnant or breastfeeding, or are on any
medications. Do not use any remedies on children under the age of 2 years
without first checking with an herbalist. Patch test any external remedies
24 hours before using to check for allergies. The author and the publishers
expressly disclaim any responsibility for loss, harm or damage from the use
or misuse of this book or your failure to seek proper medical advice.

Contents

FOREWORD
5

A CURIOUS HERBAL
6

THE HERITAGE HERBAL
14

SIMPLE PREPARATIONS
16

DIRECTORY OF HERBS & FLOWERS
20

HERBARIUM
162

INDEX
170

RESOURCES
174

ACKNOWLEDGEMENTS
176

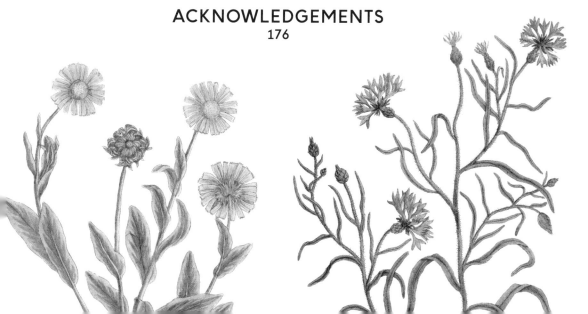

Plate 241

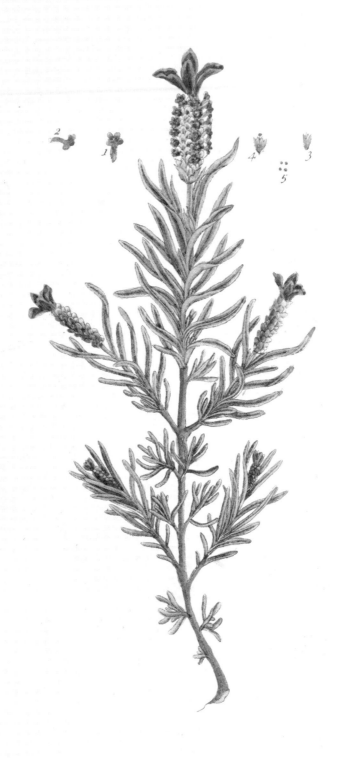

Stœchas, or *French Lavender.*

Eliz Blackwell delin. Sculp. et Pinx.

1. Flower.
2. Flower separate.
3. Calix.
4. Calix open.
5. Seed.

Stœchas arabica or purparia

FOREWORD

A wise woman once said 'you can never have too many books', but we would like to propose that 'you can never have too many herbal books', and Sonya Patel Ellis's *The Heritage Herbal* is a valuable addition to the shelves of all plant, herbal, recipe and illustration lovers alike. The use of Elizabeth Blackwell's stunning hand-coloured, whole plant etchings (1737–39) connect us with the botany and medicine of the past but Sonya also provides a delightful range of recipes that will appeal to the modern reader. This herbal gives a peek into a 'herstory' of one of the often-overlooked women in the history of herbals and healing. It also highlights the wealth of treasures contained in the British Library that provide a wonderful resource for researchers, historians or anyone interested in the world at large. Sonya has created a beautiful book that should be valued for generations to come: these richly illustrated pages are a feast for the eyes, while the recipes and remedies should satisfy the reader's body and soul.

Kim Walker & Vicky Chown
Handmade Apothecary
Authors of *The Handmade Apothecary* (2017)
and *The Herbal Remedy Handbook* (2019)

OPPOSITE: **French lavender,** *Lavandula stoechas*.

Plate 197.

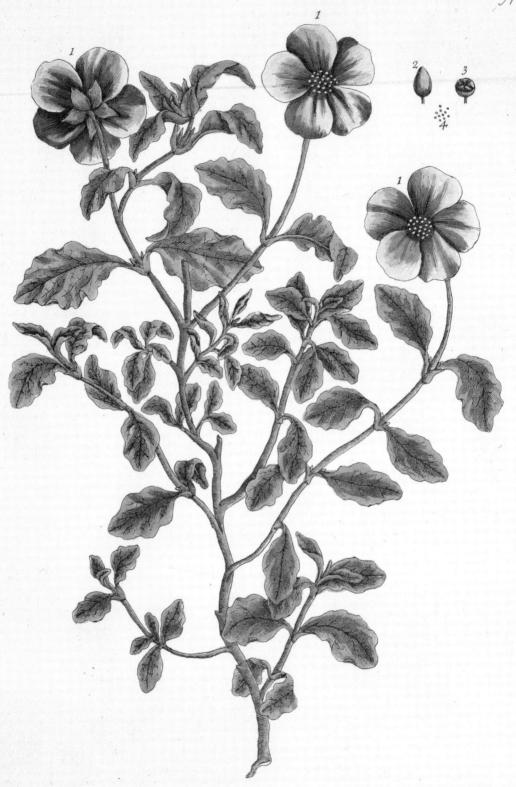

The Sweet Cistus of Candy.

Eliz. Blackwell delin. sculp. et Pinx.

1. Flower.
2. Seed Vessel.
3. Seed Vessel open.
4. Seed.

Cistus landifera vera Cretica.

A CURIOUS HERBAL

The illustrations that decorate *The Heritage Herbal* are all taken from a significant eighteenth-century publication. Not only are they useful and beautiful, they also paint a picture of a pivotal moment in the history of herbals and the life of the courageous and forward-thinking female creative behind them.

More than just a collection of herbs, herbals were once vital to the survival and expansion of civilisations around the world, evidenced by millennia-old records dating back to ancient China, Egypt, India, Persia, Greece and Rome. Elizabeth Blackwell's *A Curious Herbal* (1737–39) was no exception, helping to equip eighteenth-century communities in Britain and her colonies with essential, fully illustrated, easily identifiable knowledge of plant-based food and medicine, and raised the bar for the herbals that followed. Its publication was made all the more remarkable by Elizabeth's determination to publish a herbal for the times that would also provide funds to pay for the release of her charlatan husband from debtor's prison. It is a curious herbal in more ways than one.

In the early 1730s, this young Scottish woman set about creating a comprehensive new herbal that would bring together medicinal, edible and useful herbs from Old and New Worlds. Published originally in 125 weekly sections, the resulting two volumes (1737 and 1739) showcased over 500 plants, including herbs, fruits, vegetables, spices, tea, coffee, cotton, tobacco and several curiosities such as Mandrake – each one drawn, engraved and coloured by Elizabeth's own hand.

Not only did this work deliver a fully illustrated handbook for physicians, apothecaries and enlightened persons of the newly ratified United Kingdom, as well as a vital survival tool for British colonies in relatively unknown lands such as North America, monies received for the eventual publication of the book also secured the release of Elizabeth's wayward spouse. A modern herbal for the times, this beautifully

OPPOSITE: Rock rose, *Cistus ladanifer.*

illustrated tome also drew upon centuries of herbal history, much of which – as *The Heritage Herbal* reveals – is still relevant to this day.

Leafing through an original copy of Elizabeth's exquisitely crafted *A Curious Herbal* in the British Library is an awe-inspiring experience solely on the level of aesthetics and creative endeavour alone. Add the book's backstory of love, female determination, insightful entrepreneurship and centuries of herbal wisdom and folklore and it's surprising that Elizabeth's publication isn't subject to more pomp and grandeur in modern times.

Born between 1707 and 1713 in Aberdeen, and the daughter of a wealthy Scottish stocking merchant, Elizabeth Blackwell née Blackrie was well educated in the arts, music and languages as befit the ladies of her time. Marriage would most certainly have been on the cards. Eloping to London with a young hustler and second cousin by the name of Alexander Blackwell may not have been what her upstanding family had in mind. Indeed, the union would prove to be both Elizabeth's downfall and her making.

Alexander's father held the prestigious position of Professor of Divinity at Aberdeen's Marischal College and Blackwell was said to be something of an accomplished Greek and Latin scholar himself, yet the young buck's path was not to be paved with academic success. Although he made moves to practise as a doctor, his claims to have studied medicine under the great Dutch botanist and scientist Herman Boerhaave did not stand up. He and his young bride subsequently fled to London.

Once there, Alexander worked briefly for a publisher before setting up as a printer, although a lack of formal training would serve to be his undoing once again. Breaching trade regulations incurred hefty fines that the couple could not afford to pay, and Alexander was eventually carted off to debtor's prison. Alone in the city, Elizabeth was left to fend for herself and her young family.

Whatever the motivation – love, loyalty, desperation or a heady mix of all three – Elizabeth drew upon her own artistic talents, childhood love of botany and inherited business sense, and she concocted a plan. Discerning an opening for an up-to-date, fully illustrated reference work for apothecaries that included newly discovered plant species from North and South America in addition to the heritage herbs of the time, she set about drumming up the necessary backing for her publication.

Bolstered by the initial support of esteemed physicians Sir Hans Sloane (1660–1753) and Dr Richard Mead (1673–1754) based on the preliminary drawings of medicinal herbs she presented, Elizabeth took up lodgings at Swan Walk, in close proximity to the Chelsea Physic Garden. Established in 1673, the teaching garden of the Society of Apothecaries (itself founded in 1617) held a growing collection of plant specimens, including beneficial herbs from all over the world. It provided ample source material for her needs.

The garden's *horti praefectus* (garden director) and demonstrator of plants, the botanist and apothecary Isaac Rand (1674–1743), was also on hand to provide practical assistance and encouragement. He in turn introduced Elizabeth to Philip Miller (1691–1771), chief gardener at Chelsea and author of the highly acclaimed *The Gardener's Dictionary*, first published in 1731. Miller's book was the first published horticultural treatise that did not attach occult superstitions to plants and herbs.

If you search for copies of *A Curious Herbal* in the British Library catalogue, you will also come across a play written some 200 years later by Anne Constance Smedley. It offers a humorous, outlandish yet illuminating insight into Elizabeth's potential dealings with these two men – and the 'glasshouse' ceiling that Elizabeth had to break through to produce her herbal. Miller in particular, the play suggests, may have been harder to win round than his more encouraging counterpart Rand; curiosity in women was deemed highly unseemly at the time.

Against all the odds, Elizabeth did indeed get her herbal published, spending several years observing and drawing plants in the hallowed grounds of the Chelsea Physic Garden before arranging both the printing and promotion of her book. First issued as *A Curious Herbal, containing five hundred cuts of the most useful plants, which are now used in the practice of physick, to which is added a short description of ye plants and their common uses in Physick* in weekly parts, the first bound volume was printed by Samuel Harding in 1737, with further issues published by a bookseller known as John Nourse in 1739.

As well as engraving her own illustrations, she also set the plates for the brief yet succinct notes that accompany each herb, with text garnered from her imprisoned husband. Elizabeth also referenced the botanist

Joseph Miller's *Botanicum Officinale* (1722) and probably the Scottish anatomist and botanist Patrick Blair's *Pharmaco-Botanologia* (1723) to describe medical properties, while some plates were copied from Hendrik van Rheede tot Drakenstein's *Hortus Indicus Malabaricus* (1678–93), with due credit assigned.

Elizabeth would also have been familiar with earlier printed (post 1480) herbals and pharmacopoeias of the time such as John Gerard's *Herball*, or *General Historie of Plants* (1597), the *London Pharmacopoeia* (1618), John Parkinson's *Paradisi in Sole, Paradisus Terrestris* (1629) and Nicholas Culpeper's *The English Physician Enlarged* or *Complete Herbal* (1653), plus highly influential ancient texts such as Theophrastus' *Historia Plantarum* (350–287 BC), Dioscorides' *De Materia Medica* (AD 50–70), Pliny the Elder's *Naturalis Historia* (AD 77–79) and Avicenna's *Canon of Medicine* (1025).

Backed by the authority of the Royal College of Physicians and its governing body – the twin figures of Theophrastus and Dioscorides staring out from *A Curious Herbal*'s title page were part of the college's coat of arms – Elizabeth's work was a forerunner for William Woodville's *Medical Botany* (1790–93). With almost 300 plates drawn by renowned botanical artist James Sowerby (1757–1822), the latter became the standard illustrated work on British medicinal substances for most of the nineteenth century.

The *British Pharmacopoeia* followed suit in 1864, which in its updated form still provides the UK's official standard for pharmaceuticals today. Yet despite advances in modern medicine through the nineteenth, twentieth and twenty-first centuries, the concept of the herbal survived. Notable classics include Mrs M. Grieve's astoundingly comprehensive *A Modern Herbal* (1931) – an invaluable resource for home use during the interwar years as edited by Hilda Leyel – *Rosemary Gladstar's Herbal Recipes for Vibrant Health* (2001), and more recent publications such as Kim Walker and Vicky Chown's *The Handmade Apothecary* (2017) and Alys Fowler's *A Modern Herbal* (2019).

Various original copies of Elizabeth Blackwell's *A Curious Herbal* have also stood the test of time, several of which can be found within the

OPPOSITE: **Valerian,** *Valeriana officinalis*

Plate 250.

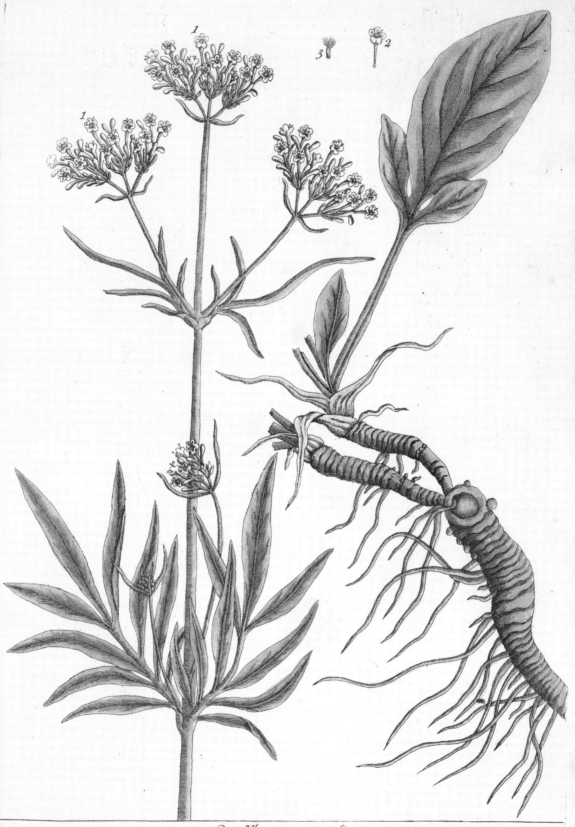

1

1

3

2

Valerian.

1. *Flower.*
2. *Flower separate.*
3. *Seed.*

Valeriana or Phu.

Eliz. Blackwell delin. sculp. et Pinx.

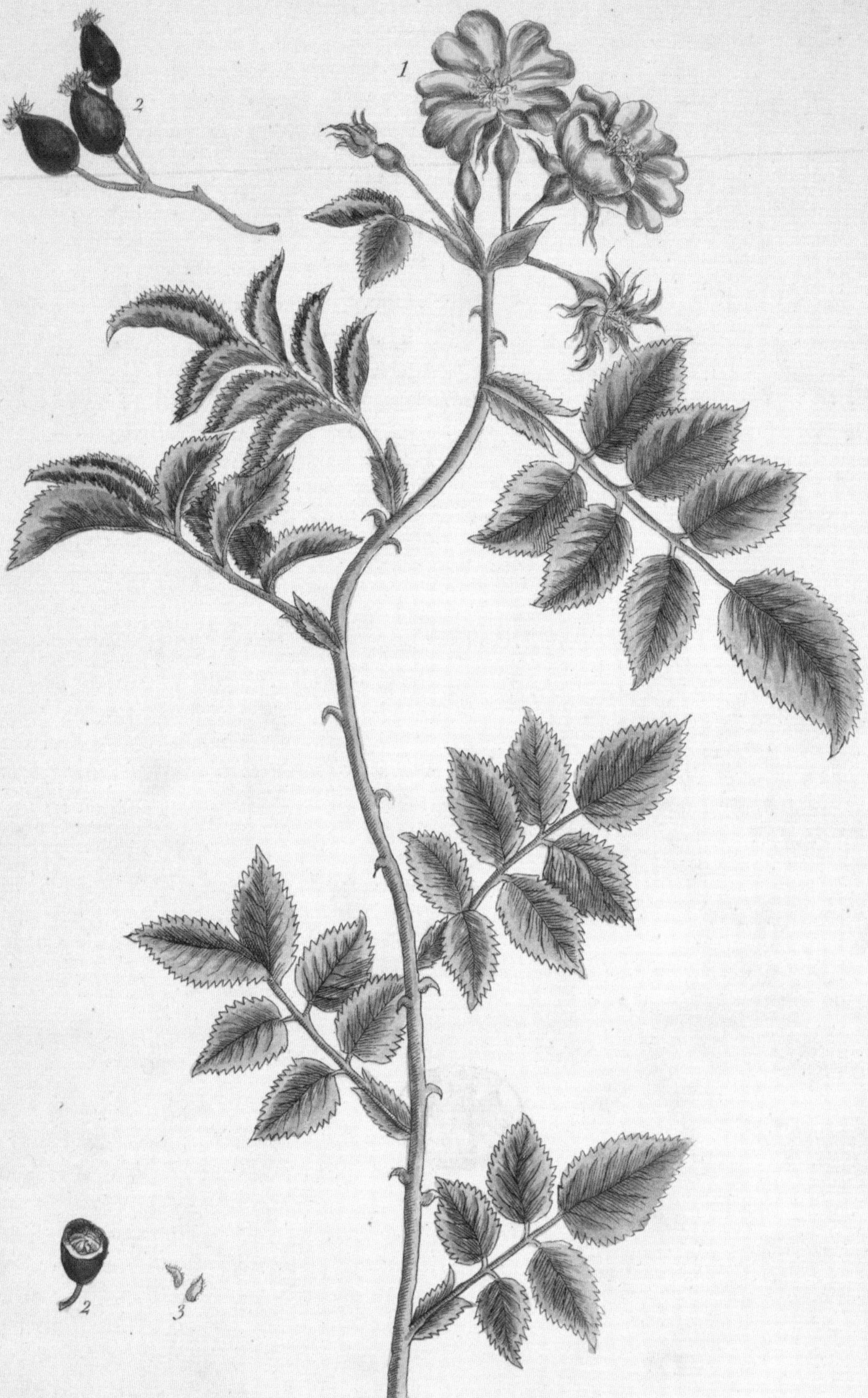

Plate 8

British Library's main catalogue and rare books archive. A 1737 hand-coloured edition belonged to the great English botanist and longstanding President of the Royal Society of London, Sir Joseph Banks (1743–1820), and includes annotations and notes on each plate including the Linnaean name for plants. *A Curious Herbal*, it should be noted, did not include Carl Linnaeus's two-part species names as part of the engraved text, as his *Species Plantarum*, the first book to officialise binomial nomenclature, was not published until 1753. The second copy was previously part of King George III's collection, and combines coloured Samuel Harding and John Nourse volumes from 1737 and 1739 respectively. While a third, produced in 1782, remains uncoloured, offering a different perspective on each herb.

Although 48 pages of *A Curious Herbal* have been made accessible as a virtual book using the British Library's unique Turning the Pages™ technology, *The Heritage Herbal* is unique in bringing so many of Elizabeth's wonderful illustrations to life in print, including some of the most beautiful flowering herbs such as calendula, cornflower, fennel, rose, rock rose and saffron and all of the most enduring ones such as chamomile, lavender, sage, thyme and rosemary. Make an appointment to view one of the Library's rare editions, or peruse an illustrated version of *A Curious Herbal* online (see Resources, pages 174–175) and you will also find illustrations of fruits, vegetables, nuts, spices and the high-value commodities tea, coffee and cotton.

The Heritage Herbal pays homage to the use of herbs both past and present and honours the memory of the utterly devoted and ingenious Elizabeth Blackwell, who did indeed manage to fund her husband's release from jail. Alexander was, however, later executed for alleged treason on the orders of his employer at the time, the King of Sweden. This book was also written in celebration of a woman who, despite the odds, used her passion and artistic talent, love of plants and sheer willpower to bring a plan to fruition – a female force present in every carefully observed, hand-drawn leaf, stalk, petal, flower and seed of this book.

Sonya Patel Ellis

OPPOSITE: **Dog rose, *Rosa canina*.**

THE HERITAGE HERBAL

Gathering together herbal history from ancient works to more modern tomes, *The Heritage Herbal*'s Directory of Herbs & Flowers uses a heritage format of 'description', 'name', 'time', 'place' and 'virtues' to communicate past and present uses of 35 selected herbs. This *modus operandi* was employed by historic herbalists John Gerard, Nicholas Culpeper and John Parkinson and, in looser form, Elizabeth Blackwell, delivering at-a-glance information about identifying, gathering, growing, eating, healing and crafting with herbs.

Each entry in this book also includes practical remedies and recipes to heal, nourish and style (see opposite), some of them developed from simple preparations (see pages 16–17) passed down the centuries, others that signify the most pertinent application of a particular herb or the most apt use for modern-day living. Many of these recipes and remedies can also be adapted to suit individual preferences or tastes – swapping sugar for honey or sweet almond oil for coconut oil, for example, using dried herbs instead of fresh ones, or making bigger or smaller batches to store, gift or test out.

Organised in alphabetical order according to botanical name, from *Angelica archangelica* (angelica) to *Viola tricolor* (viola heartsease), it's also easy to pinpoint a herb by its common name via the directory contents on pages 20–21. Turn to the handy Herbarium of themed uses at the back of the book for further inspiration regarding specific medicinal properties, flavour or texture, crafting potential, or the ornamental value of herbs. The more familiar herbs become, the more useful they can be.

On a final note, read through each recipe in full before commencing to ensure that you have all relevant tools and materials to hand, as well as the ingredients. Some recipes require specialist equipment such as a blender, grinder, funnel, strainer or non-reactive pan, while many need one or several sterilised containers in which to prepare and store herbs (see page 17). Working with herbs can be a real, beneficial pleasure so give yourself time and permission to slow down and enjoy the process.

HERBS TO GROW AND GATHER

People have been growing and gathering herbs for millennia, for pleasure and for purpose, and to heal, nourish and style their lives. It is possible to forage for some herbs in the wild but make sure you have permission (see page 16) and seek expert advice if you are unsure about a species. Growing your own herbs can bring peace of mind on the identification front, a ready harvest and some multi-sensory beauty to a garden or windowsill. For inspiration on what to grow, see the Herbarium on pages 162–3. For more specific advice on growing and gathering herbs, visit the individual entries in the Directory.

HERBS TO HEAL

Before the advent of modern medicine, herbals were a vital way of delivering everyday healing and healthcare. Many of the health-boosting, medicinal plant properties that these herbals describe are now supported by scientific research, from the power of lavender's essential oils to the skin-soothing potential of calendula. Consult the Herbarium on pages 164–5 as a holistic health and wellbeing guide. For more specific recipes and remedies to heal, visit the individual herb entries in the Directory.

HERBS TO NOURISH

Herbs have been used to flavour, scent, texture and garnish food for centuries, in some cases providing the main ingredient for a dish or a vital nutritional staple in hard times or while moving from place to place. Today, many of these herbs have been scientifically proven to be rich in beneficial vitamins, minerals and flavonoids, as well as being highly aromatic, flavoursome or beautifying. Use the Herbarium on pages 166–7 as a culinary guide. For more specific recipes and remedies to nourish, visit the individual herb entries in the Directory.

HERBS TO STYLE

Herbals were primarily created to promote the nutritional and medicinal value of herbs, but such aromatic and often attractive plants were also traditionally used to beautify, inspire, perfume and decorate both body and home, with many of these uses handed down and recorded for posterity. Use the Herbarium on pages 168–9 as a creative and inspirational guide to enhance your lifestyle. For more specific recipes and ideas to style, visit the individual herb entries in the Directory.

SIMPLE PREPARATIONS

Herbals, ancient and modern, have been made even more useful by the inclusion of simple preparations, such as herbal infusions, decoctions, oils, syrups, vinegars, poultices and salves alongside directories of medicinal and culinary herbs. These 'simples', some of which appear overleaf, have then been adapted through the ages to create more pertinent preparations. Many of these form the basis of the recipes and remedies in the Directory of Herbs & Flowers.

Harvesting Herbs

The best way to harvest herbs differs between species. There are, however, a few basic rules, which can help ensure that plants and people stay healthy and happy along the way.

❧ Know what you're picking – some plants can be poisonous or harmful under certain conditions when ingested or touched. If in doubt, consult an expert guide.

❧ Wear gloves if necessary (see Nettle, page 150) and always wash hands and herbs after gathering to remove dirt, unwanted substances or bugs.

❧ Only harvest one third of a plant at a time; chives and lavender are exceptions.

❧ Pinch leafy annual herbs such as basil at the tips of stems, gathering several leaves at a time.

❧ Cut longer stemmed herbs such as coriander, parsley, lavender and rosemary near the base.

❧ Harvest sprigs of perennial herbs such as oregano, thyme, sage and tarragon.

❧ Many herbs are at their best just before flowering, others when the plant reaches a certain height or maturity. Harvesting edible flowers, seeds or nutritious roots depends on the season. Consult the Directory for advice on individual herbs.

Foraging

When foraging for herbs, ensure that you follow the relevant countryside code or law. In the UK this means: asking permission to forage on private property from the landowner or occupier; never removing rare or protected plants or roots from common land; only picking for personal use; and only picking from plentiful populations and not too much of any given plant. Also avoid polluted spots. Find useful resources on page 175.

Storing Herbs

There are several ways to store herbs including freezing, drying and preserving in oil, vinegar, sugar or salt. Follow these simple tips:

❧ Freshly picked herbs should be washed and patted dry, unless the recipe or remedy states otherwise. Continue to wear gloves while handling any irritant herbs (see Nettle page 150).

❧ Herbs with low moisture content such as marjoram, oregano, rosemary, summer savory and thyme can be air-dried. Harvest before flowering, mid-morning when the dew has dried but before they wilt in the afternoon sun. Remove damaged leaves, shake off insects, tie 4–6 stems together with twine and hang upside down in a warm dry place for around 2 weeks. Place herb bundles in a perforated paper bag first to collect loose matter. Herbs should be dry enough to crumble before placing in an airtight jar to store. Use within 1 year.

❧ Herbs with succulent leaves or a higher moisture content such as basil, chives, mint or tarragon can be dried using a dehydrator, or preserved in the freezer. Place gently cleaned stems in bags first, or combine with water or oil in ice cube trays to use one portion at a time.

Preparing Herbs & Recipes

❧ Use fresh or dried herbs as specified in ingredients lists or recipes. In some cases, fresh and dried herbs are interchangeable. The quantities of herb, however, will need to be adjusted, as advised, as the potency of dried herbs can often be twice that of fresh ones.

❧ Wash your hands before preparing herbs and avoid touching eyes or mouth while following a recipe, unless specified. Some herbs can be toxic or irritating to the skin in their raw state.

❧ Don't be tempted to skip the sterilisation stage for storage containers or other specified tools or equipment. This helps to avoid contaminating produce with harmful bacteria, yeasts, fungi or other organisms, and reducing shelf life. Choose from oven, water immersion, dishwasher or microwave methods of sterilisation depending on the material. Glass containers can generally be washed with warm soapy water, rinsed and placed in a low oven (140°C/280°F) for 15–20 minutes; soak lids and rubber seals in boiling water. To avoid breakages, ensure that the container you are using is the same temperature as the produce you are placing in it: hot in hot and cold in cold.

RIGHT: **Yarrow**, *Achillea millefolium*.

Stay Safe

Avoid adjusting quantities of herbs or essential oils in recipes, especially in medicinal preparations. Too much could impede or counteract any healing effects or flavour. In some cases, it could even prove harmful to health. Some herbs, herbal preparations or ingredients, such as essential oils, can be harmful for children, pregnant women or those with a medical condition. Always read the advisory notes and consult a doctor if unsure.

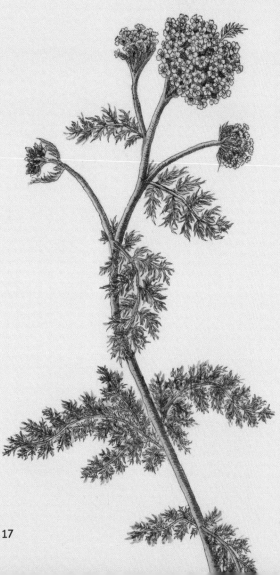

Herbal Infusion

Steep tender leaves, flowers or buds such as chamomile, mint, jasmine, nettle, thyme, sage, lemon balm, tarragon and viola heartsease in just boiled water to create a soothing herbal infusion to drink as tea or use in specific remedies or recipes. Infusing rather than boiling or simmering can help preserve precious vitamins, essential oils and enzymes.

Makes around 1 litre (1 quart)

4–6 tbsp dried or 6–8 tbsp fresh leaves, flowers, buds, berries, seeds (or other aromatic parts)

1 litre (1 quart) just-boiled water

1 Place the dried or freshly picked herbs in a 1 litre (1 quart) glass jar. Cover with the water and leave to steep for up to 30–40 minutes. Check specific herbs for recommended times – some infusions are ready in 5–10 minutes.

2 Strain through a fine mesh sieve or muslin into a clean, sterilised jar (compost used herbs).

3 Serve by the cup or use as desired, discarding after 1–2 days.

4 Alternatively, make a solar infusion by placing herbs in cold water in a clean, sterilised jar set in a sunny spot. Leave for several hours, then strain and use as above.

Herbal Decoction

Extract the active constituents of roots, bark, twiggy elements and some seeds and nuts by gently simmering in a pan of boiling water. This works well for herbs such as chicory or angelica root, dried elderberries or fennel seeds.

Makes 1 litre (1 quart)

4–6 tbsp dried or 6–8 tbsp fresh fibrous or woody plant parts, such as roots, bark, twiggy parts and some seeds and nuts

1 Place the dried or fresh plant parts in a non-reactive pan and add 1 litre (1 quart) water. Bring to a boil and then simmer gently for 25–45 minutes, depending on strength required.

2 Strain through a fine mesh sieve or muslin into a clean, sterilised jar (compost used herbs).

3 Serve by the cup or use as desired, discarding after 1–2 days. For a stronger decoction, cover and leave to infuse overnight.

Herbal Infused Oil

❧ Infused oils are a lovely way to capture the power of herbs with high levels of volatile oils, or those with fat soluble components such as basil, oregano, rosemary, calendula, peppermint, rose or lavender.

❧ Choose food-grade olive oil or coconut oil for edible concoctions, or sweet almond

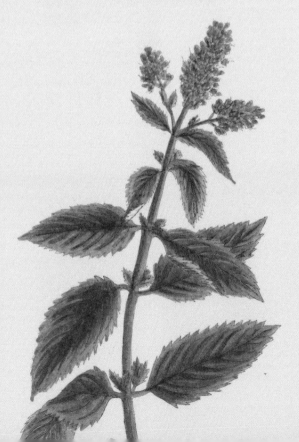

LEFT: Peppermint, *Mentha* x *piperita*.

or jojoba carrier oil for baths, massages or salves.

Makes around 500ml (17½fl oz)
Handful of chosen herbs, ideally as dry as possible
Suitable food-grade or cosmetic vegetable oil such as olive, coconut, sweet almond or jojoba oil

1 Chop the herbs and place in a double boiler or a bowl over a pan of boiling water. Cover with 2.5–5cm (1–2in) of preferred oil. Heat on a slow simmer for 30–60 minutes, checking to ensure the oil doesn't overheat.

2 Remove from the heat when golden or golden-green, with a beautifully fragrant or aromatic smell. Strain through a muslin cloth into a clean, sterilised airtight 500ml (17½fl oz) glass jar. Allow to cool before use.

3 Alternatively, make a solar infused oil by filling a clean, sterilised airtight jar half full with chosen herbs and covering fully with oil. Leave in a warm, sunny spot for up to 2 weeks. Replenish herbs and repeat before straining into a fresh sterilised jar.

Herbal Infused Syrup

Syrups are generally cooked-down, concentrated herbal infusions or decoctions with added sweetener such as sugar or honey – ideal for sore throats, helping some less palatable medicines go down, or to use in desserts, puddings or cocktails. Try using elderberries, thyme, marjoram, saffron, sweet violet or rose.

Makes around 1 litre (1 quart)
1 litre (1 quart) herbal infusion or decoction (see above)
125–250g (1–2 cups) brown sugar or 350–700g (1–2 cups) honey, to taste

1 Place the herbal infusion or decoction in a pan and gently simmer until reduced by half to around 500ml (17½fl oz). If making from scratch, remember to strain out any herbs.

2 Stir in the sugar or honey and add more if sweeter syrup is desired. Warm over a low heat until fully combined.

3 Allow to cool a little, then decant into a 1 litre (1 quart) sterilised airtight glass jar. Store in the fridge for up to 3 months.

More Simple Preparations to Try, Adapt & Gift

❧ Make a cooling or perfuming flower water or hydrosol – see rose (page 116), and cornflower (page 44).

❧ Create a soothing or healing salve or poultice – see lavender (page 80), salad burnet (page 136) and savory (page 140).

❧ Prepare a medicinal or culinary vinegar or oxymel – see chervil (page 28) and hyssop (page 72).

❧ Concoct a medicinal herbal tincture – see sage (page 128).

❧ Find simple recipes for homemade soaps or bath bombs – see calendula (page 40) or cornflower (page 45).

❧ Herbal salts and sugars make lovely culinary or therapeutic gifts – see lavender (page 81).

❧ Herbal cordials have stood the test of time to refresh and invigorate – see elderflower (page 133) and tarragon (page 33).

For specific remedies and recipes see the Directory of Herbs & Flowers starting on page 22.

DIRECTORY OF HERBS & FLOWERS

ANGELICA *Angelica archangelica*   22

CHERVIL *Anthriscus cerefolium*   26

TARRAGON *Artemisia dracunculus*   30

BORAGE *Borago officinalis*   34

CALENDULA *Calendula officinalis*   38

CORNFLOWER *Centaurea cyanus*   42

CHAMOMILE *Chamaemelum nobile*   46

CHICORY *Cichorium intybus*   50

CORIANDER *Coriandrum sativum*   54

SAFFRON *Crocus sativus*   58

FENNEL *Foeniculum vulgare*   62

LIQUORICE *Glycyrrhiza glabra*   66

HYSSOP *Hyssopus officinalis*   70

JASMINE *Jasminum officinale*   74

LAVENDER *Lavendula*   78

LOVAGE *Levisticum officinale*   82

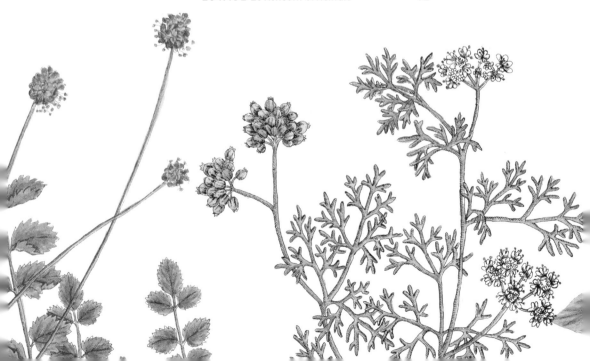

LEMON BALM *Melissa officinalis*   86

MINT *Mentha*   90

SWEET CICELY *Myrrhis odorata*   94

BASIL *Ocimum basilicum*   98

MARJORAM *Origanum majorana*   102

OREGANO *Origanum vulgare*   106

PARSLEY *Petroselinum crispum*   110

ROSE *Rosa*   114

ROSEMARY *Rosmarinus officinalis*   118

SORREL *Rumex*   122

SAGE *Salvia officinalis*   126

ELDER *Sambucus nigra*   130

SALAD BURNET *Sanguisorba minor*   134

SAVORY *Satureja*   138

DANDELION *Taraxacum officinale*   142

THYME *Thymus*   146

NETTLE *Urtica dioica*   150

SWEET VIOLET *Viola odorata*   154

VIOLA HEARTSEASE *Viola tricolor*   158

ANGELICA
Angelica archangelica, Apiaceae family

This tall, earthy 'Viking herb' biennial with purplish-green stems and greenish-yellow umbels was regarded as a virtuous cure-all for much of the past two millennia. Indeed 'Angelica, the garden kinde, is so good an herbe,' mused John Parkinson in *Paradisi in Sole, Paradisus Terrestris* (1629), 'that there is no part thereof but is of much use ... whether you will distill the water of the herbe, or preserve or candie the rootes or the greene stalkes, or use the seeds in powder or in distillations, or deceptions with other things.' Today, we know it as a large, aromatic garden ornamental, and for its bright green, candied stalks.

❧ THE DESCRIPTION Plants grow to 1.5–2.5 metres (5–8 feet) tall, with fluted (grooved) and hollow, pink-tinted, celery-tasting stalks rising from a thick brown taproot, handsome pinnately or palmately divided leaves up the stem, and large globular umbels of yellow-green flowers that bear pale yellow fruits. To be safe, grow your own to avoid mistaking for toxic family relatives such as hemlock (*Conium maculatum*).

❧ THE NAME According to one legend laid out by Mrs M. Grieve in *A Modern Herbal* (1931), 'Angelica was revealed in a dream by an angel to cure the plague'. She also relates 'that it blooms on the day of Michael the Archangel ... and is on that account a preservative against evil spirits and witchcraft'. Indeed, angelica was held in such high esteem it was widely nicknamed 'The Root of the Holy Ghost'.

❧ THE PLACE *Angelica archangelica* (garden angelica) is one of around 60 species of *Angelica* including *Angelica sylvestris* (wild angelica) and *Angelica sinensis* (Chinese *dong quai*). It grows wild in northern Scandinavia, Russia, Iceland, Greenland and the Faroe Islands, and has been cultivated in Western Europe since the 10th century. It prefers a cool climate, moist well-drained soil, a sunny spot where its roots will be in shade and plenty of space.

❧ THE TIME *A Modern Herbal* (1931) advises that 'The root should be dug up in the autumn of the first year' to avoid mould and insect damage. The plant produces its tall flowering stems after its second year and cutting off early summer flower heads before they set seed, while harvesting the tender hollow stalks can encourage short-lived perennial behaviour. Sow ripe seeds and transplant young seedlings in early autumn.

❧ THE VIRTUES Historically used in powder, syrup, poultice or infusion form to treat ailments and infections such as 'wind', 'the biting of a mad dog', 'old filfy deep ulcers' (Nicholas Culpeper, *Complete Herbal*, 1653) and 'the Plague' (John Gerard, *Herball*, 1597), garden angelica has also traditionally been used in confectionery and preserves. It is now known to be carminative (helps prevent gas), expectorant (mucus-discharging) and diaphoretic (induces perspiration).

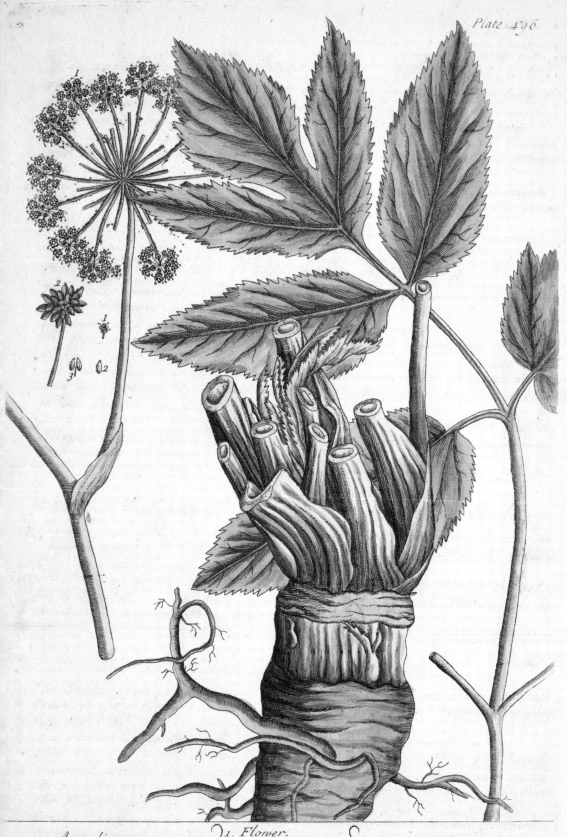

Plate 496.

Angelica.

Eliz. Blackwell delin. sculp. et Pinx.

} 1. Flower. {
} 2. Seed Veſſel. {
} 3. Seed Veſſel separate. {

Angelica.

HEAL
ANGELICA ROOT TEA

Try bitter, warming and invigorating angelica tea to treat poor circulation or digestive issues. The flavour is also traditionally thought to dispel the urge for alcohol – ironic considering that angelica is a key component of gin, vermouth and Chartreuse liqueur. Avoid if pregnant, using blood-thinning drugs, or if diabetic.

Makes 250ml (1 cup)
250ml (1 cup) boiling water
1 tsp fresh (crushed) or dried angelica root

1 Place the root in the boiling water.

2 Steep for 5–15 minutes.

3 Drink a cupful twice daily for the most warming or digestive effects.

Other uses
❧ Place crushed angelica leaves in the home or car to freshen the air or help ward off motion sickness.
❧ Blend sweet almond oil with angelica seed essential oil for a fortifying massage.

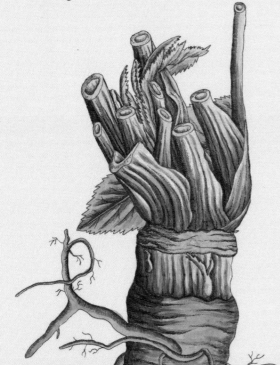

NOURISH
ANGELICA JAM

Contemporary recipes for turning angelica stems into jam often add lemon juice, lemon rind or half-parts rhubarb to give the earthiness some tang – the end result being something like gin-flavoured jam.

Makes 3 x 450g (1lb) jars
1kg (2lb 4oz) angelica stems
700g (1.5lb) granulated sugar
Zest and juice of 1 lemon

1 Cut the tender stems of angelica into fairly long strips.

2 Pre-cook by blanching in simmering water until soft. This can take up to 30 minutes. Transfer to a bowl of cold water and leave to soak for 12 hours. Strain and cut into small chunks.

3 Place the angelica, sugar and 425ml (1¾ cups) water in a pan and heat slowly. Stir continuously until the sugar is dissolved.

4 Add the lemon juice and rind and bring to the boil until jam setting point of 110°C (230°F) is reached. Test by dropping 1 tsp onto a chilled plate; it should wrinkle slightly when touched.

5 Cool slightly, pour into three warm, sterilised 450g (1lb) jam jars and immediately seal with lids.

6 Serve your 'gin' jam on warm toast.

Other uses
❧ Dry homegrown angelica seeds in a dehydrator or a low oven, then grind to use in baking or roasts.
❧ Harvest fresh tender angelica stalks in spring or from low growth in summer and sauté in butter.

STYLE
TUTTI FRUTTI ICE CREAM

Old preserving books almost always include a recipe for candied or crystallised angelica, as a way to conserve the herb. Once a popular decoration for cakes and desserts, candied angelica is also the emerald-green component of traditional tutti frutti ice cream.

Serves 8–10
For the candied stems:
100g (3.5oz) tender angelica stems
200g (1 cup) granulated sugar
**   (plus extra for tossing)**

For the tutti frutti ice cream:
2 egg whites
110g (½ cup) white caster sugar
300ml (10fl oz) double or whipping cream
1 tsp vanilla extract
60g (2oz) candied angelica (see above)
60g (2oz) candied pineapple
60g (2oz) natural glacé cherries

1 Strip the stems of the leaves. Cut into 7cm (3in) lengths. Blanch in simmering water for 15 seconds. Place in a bowl.

2 Combine the sugar and 250ml (1 cup) of water in a separate pan. Bring to the boil until syrupy. Pour over the stems. Cover and chill for 12 hours. Repeat twice, then remove the stems and blot dry.

3 Dehydrate the stems in a low oven (40°C/100°F) for around 4 hours, or in a warm, dry place for several days. Cool, toss in sugar and set to one side.

4 Whisk the egg whites until stiff. Sprinkle in half the caster sugar. Whisk again. Fold in the remaining caster sugar.

5 Whisk the cream in another bowl until it thickens. Gently fold in the egg white, vanilla extract, candied angelica and pineapple and glacé cherries.

6 Spoon the mixture into a lidded tub, cover tightly and freeze for 4–6 hours until firm. Or churn in an ice-cream maker for 45 minutes.

7 Serve in bowls with small wafers or in cones.

Other uses
❧ Burn dried angelica root to help ward off negative energy in the home.
❧ Use angelica flowers, leaves or stems (as straws) in gin cocktails.

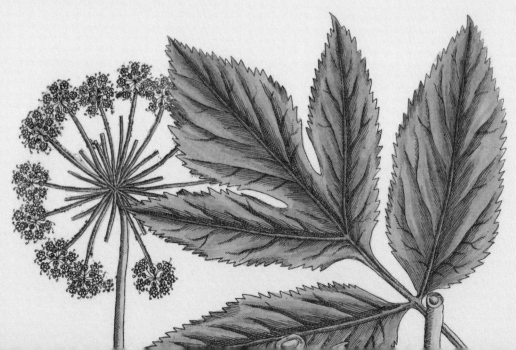

CHERVIL
Anthriscus cerefolium, Apiaceae family

White-flowered chervil, a traditional culinary herb, has often been confused with other members of the same botanical family – not only parsley (*Petroselinum crispum*), cow parsley (*Anthriscus sylvestris*) and sweet-tasting sweet cicely (*Myrrhis odorata* – see page 94), but also toxic hemlock (*Conium maculatum*). A traditional ingredient of the French herb mix *fines herbes*, the leaves of this vitamin-rich 'herb of joy' are also used to add colour and flavour to sauces and go particularly well with eggs.

❧ **THE DESCRIPTION** A somewhat petite version of flat-leaf parsley, with a mild, sweet aniseed flavour, this upright annual or biennial grows about 30–60cm (12–24in) tall, has feathery, aromatic foliage and tiny delicate flowers that form umbels before bearing oblong-ovoid 1cm (1/3in) long, beaked fruits. To avoid mistaken identity, grow chervil at home or go foraging with an expert.

❧ **THE NAME** *Anthriscus* is thought to relate to the Greek *Anthriskon* and the Latin *Anthriscus*, which were ancient names for chervil or a chervil-like plant. The species name, *cerefolium*, meaning 'waxy-leaved' or 'leaves of joy' from the ancient Latin *Chaerophyllum* – alluding to this pretty herb's shiny leaves – has been carried forward from chervil's previous name *Scandix cerefolium* attributed by Swedish botanist Carl Linnaeus in 1753.

❧ **THE PLACE** Native to the Caucasus region and western Asia, chervil is thought to have been spread throughout Europe by the Romans. Cultivated for centuries, it prefers a sheltered area with dappled shade in summer. It also fares well under deciduous trees, in pots or on an indoor windowsill out of direct sun. Grow as a companion plant next to radishes, broccoli or lettuce to deter slugs and snails.

❧ **THE TIME** Nicholas Culpeper (*Complete Herbal*, 1653) describes chervil as having a small and long root that 'perisheth every year', which 'must be sown in spring for seed, and after July for autumn sallad' and 'sown again at the end of the summer'. For the most flavoursome leaves, harvest about six to eight weeks after planting, plus pick leaves in the morning before any dehydration occurs. Chervil is best eaten fresh.

❧ **THE VIRTUES** John Gerard (*Herball*, 1597) speaks of 'good, wholesome and pleasant' leaves that 'rejoiceth and comforteth the heart', being 'very good for people that are dull and without courage'. Chervil was also used as a folk remedy for curing hiccups, 'to dissolve congealed or clotted blood in the body' (Culpeper, 1653) and for ailments of the kidneys. Today it is chervil's gourmet anise taste that has ensured its popularity.

Plate 236.

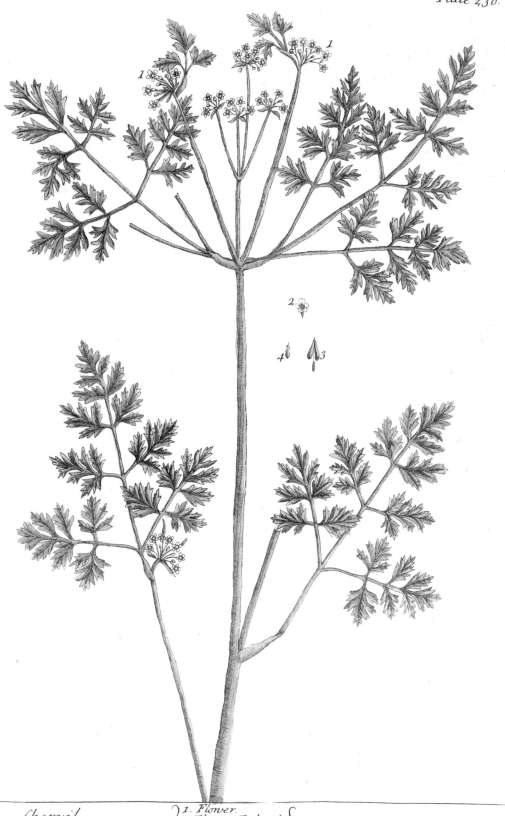

Chervil.

Eliz. Blackwell delin. sculp. et Pinx.

1. Flower.
2. Flower Enlarg'd.
3. Seed Vessel open.
4. Seed.

Chaerefolium.

HEAL
HERB OF JOY VINEGAR

Chervil's 'leaves of joy' were traditionally chewed as a restorative, especially on Maundy Thursday at the end of Lent. Preserve the sentiment along with chervil's rich supply of vitamin C, carotene, iron and magnesium by infusing vinegar with freshly plucked anise-tasting leaves – ideal as a restorative daily tonic or to freshen up salad dressings.

Makes 1 x 500ml (17½fl oz) jar
Bunch (1 cup) fresh chervil
500ml (2 cups) white wine vinegar

1 Place the chervil in a 500ml (17½fl oz) sterilised, airtight glass jar.

2 Cover with vinegar and leave to steep for 1 week.

3 Strain the infused vinegar into a jug and return to the washed and re-sterilised jar.

Other uses
❧ Help combat wrinkles with an antioxidant facemask of chopped chervil, yogurt and apple cider vinegar.
❧ Boost circulation and detoxify with a cup of chervil-infused tea.

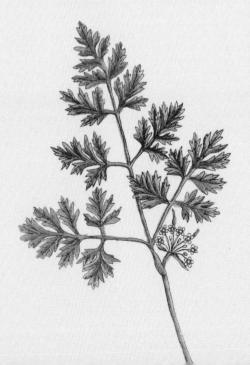

NOURISH
CHERVIL MAYONNAISE

Deliver the delicate anise taste of chervil via a creamy dip of homemade mayonnaise – perfect swirled through a new potato salad or as a dip for grilled asparagus. Garnish with an extra sprinkling of chopped fresh chervil leaves for an additional pop of spring green.

Makes 1 x 300ml (10fl oz) jar
2 large egg yolks
2 tbsp lemon juice or white wine vinegar
300ml (1¼ cups) olive oil
1 tbsp Dijon mustard
2 tsp finely chopped fresh chervil

1 Place the egg yolks in a bowl and whisk with 1 tbsp of the lemon juice or vinegar.

2 Slowly and steadily pour in the olive oil, whisking until absorbed.

3 Add the remaining lemon juice or vinegar to taste.

4 Whisk in the Dijon mustard and chervil.

5 Spoon into a sterilized, airtight 300ml (10fl oz) jar and keep in the fridge for up to 1 week.

Other uses
❧ Sprinkle chervil leaves over roasted fennel to add an extra layer of anise flavour.
❧ Make an earthy green chervil soup with shallots, celery, egg yolks, butter, stock and double cream.

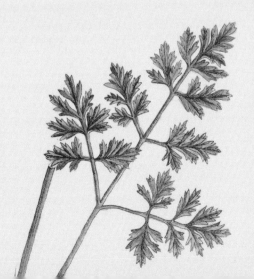

STYLE
A BOX OF *FINES HERBES*

Grow your own *fines herbes*, the classic French combination of tarragon, chervil, chives and parsley. Scatter freshly gathered herbs in equal parts on eggs or salad, or use in a *beurre blanc* sauce. These are also lovely houseplants for a windowsill out of direct sun.

For 1 trough of herbs
Large wooden trough (big enough for the 4 plant pots)
Waterproof sheet or bag
Small pot or plug plant each of chervil, tarragon, chives and parsley
16 small crocks (broken pots or small stones)
4 terracotta or ceramic plant pots 20cm (8in) diameter by 15cm (6in) deep with drainage holes and saucers
Small bag peat-free compost

1 Line the bottom and sides of a wooden trough with a waterproof sheet or bag.

2 Gently remove the plants or plugs from their pot or tray and remove any dead or damaged foliage. Place 4 crocks in the bottom of each terracotta or ceramic pot. Half-fill the pots with peat-free compost, insert a herb into each and top up with more compost.

3 Water well, letting any excess drain away; then put the pots on their saucers and position in the trough, leaving enough room for growth and spread.

4 Set the trough in a semi-sunny spot and water regularly, especially in warm weather.

Other uses
❧ Plant shade-tolerant, slug deterring chervil near radishes for an extra spicy flavour.
❧ Press delicate white chervil flowers and mount against a dark background in resin or glass domed cabochons.

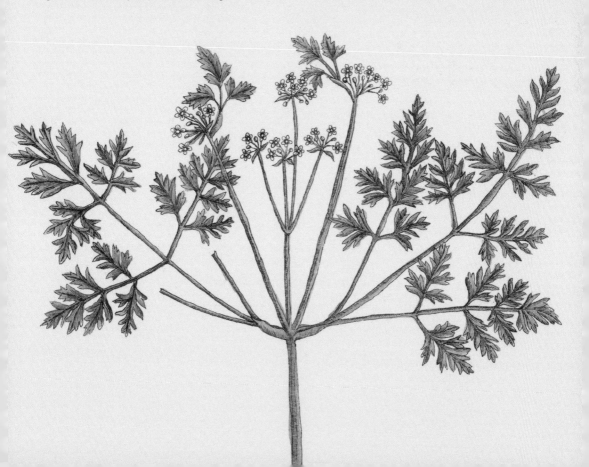

TARRAGON
Artemisia dracunculus, Asteraceae family

Slender-branched, lance-leaved and rarely flowering, tarragon is best known as a culinary herb with a flavour reminiscent of anise. Most widely used is the strong-tasting French or true tarragon (*Artemisia dracunculus* var. *sativa*) popular in béarnaise sauce and the herb mix *fines herbes*, and also used as a digestive. Russian tarragon (*A. dracunculus* var. *inodora* or *A. dracunculoides*) has a more subtle flavour, while unrelated Mexican tarragon (*Tagetes lucida*) tastes similar but is actually a type of marigold.

♣ THE DESCRIPTION Just one of hundreds of species in the diverse *Artemisia* genus, tarragon is a woody herb related to the absinthe ingredient wormwood (*A. absinthium*) and common mugwort (*A. vulgaris*). Half-hardy French tarragon has smooth, dark green, silver-sheened leaves and insignificant flowers that only set seed in warm climes. Hardy Russian tarragon has coarser leaves and tiny sprays of yellow flowers.

♣ THE NAME 'The name Tarragon is a corruption of the French *Esdragon*, derived from the Latin *Dracunculus* (a little dragon), which also serves as its specific name' (Mrs M. Grieve, *A Modern Herbal*, 1931). This 'dragon' refers to tarragon's use as an ancient remedy for serpent bites or from its snakelike roots. Its current genus name *Artemisia* stems from Artemis, an ancient queen or a Greek goddess associated with wild animals and nature, the moon, fertility and hunting.

♣ THE PLACE Tarragon is found all over temperate Eurasia and North America where it grows in a wide variety of habitats from desert shrub to sub-alpine woods. Grow in poor or fertile well-drained soil in full sun, in borders, pots or as a companion plant to most vegetables. It can also be grown in a sunny spot indoors, ideally alongside other ingredients of *fines herbes* (see page 29).

♣ THE TIME Grow French tarragon from softwood or root cuttings as it rarely produces seeds. Russian tarragon can be propagated from seed in spring. Harvest leaves of both in spring and summer, pinching off blooms for a constant supply of foliage. Bring French tarragon indoors or protect the crown with fleece over winter.

♣ THE VIRTUES 'Tarragon is hot and dry in the third degree, and not to be eaten alone in sallades, but joined with other herbs, as Lettuce, Purslain, and such like that, that it may also temper the coldness of them', advises John Gerard (*Herball*, 1597). Today tarragon is chiefly used to add a sweet, anise-like flavour to food or drinks, as a digestive, or as a deodorising essential oil.

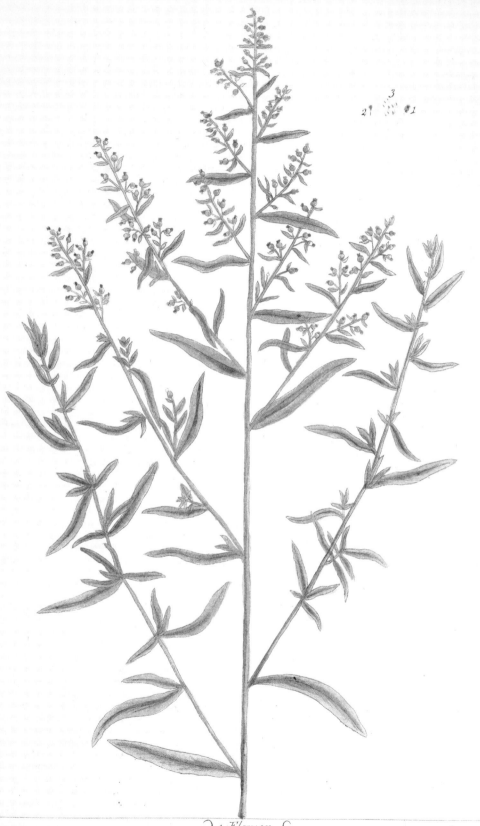

Plate 116.

3
2   1

Tarragon.   ⎰ 1. Flower ⎱   *Dracunculus hortensis.*
Eliz. Blackwell delin. sculp. et Pinx.   ⎱ 2. Fruit ⎰
                               ⎰ 3. Seed ⎱

HEAL
DIGESTIVE TARRAGON TEA

Naturally digestive tarragon, delivered as an infusion of the fresh or dry herb, can help soothe stomach pain and bloating. This is especially helpful at the end of meals. Tarragon tea is also useful as an appetite stimulant or stressbuster.

Makes 250ml (1 cup)
1 tbsp fresh or 1 tsp dried tarragon leaves
250ml (1 cup) just-boiled water

1 Steep the leaves in the just-boiled water for 5 minutes.
2 Strain the infused tea into a clean cup and drink while warm.

Other uses
❧ Sprigs of tarragon were traditionally chewed to treat tooth pain – the inherent compound eugenol is now known to have a numbing effect.
❧ Add a few drops of tarragon essential oil to an aromatherapy diffuser to help deodorise and scent the air.

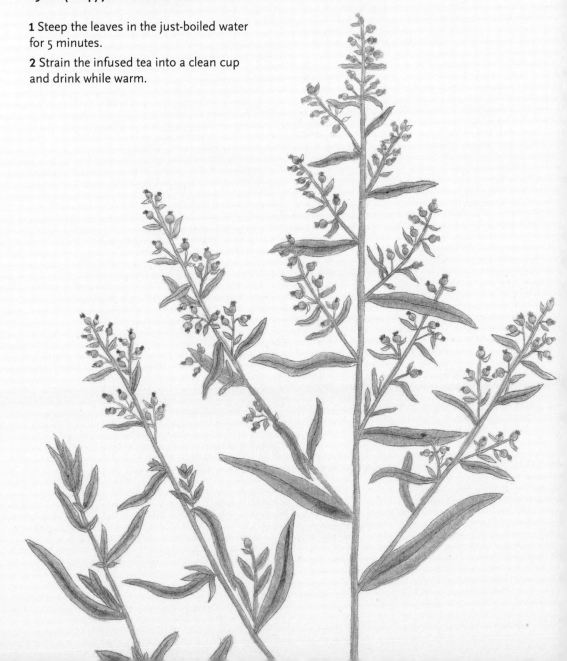

NOURISH
BÉARNAISE SAUCE

Creamy yellow béarnaise sauce gets its acidity from a vinegar and white wine reduction, flavoured by sweet tarragon, shallots, white peppercorns and cayenne pepper. Serve with eggs or grilled asparagus.

Makes 4–6 servings
4 shallots
4 white peppercorns
4 large egg yolks
225g (8oz) unsalted butter
2 tbsp chopped fresh tarragon leaves
4 tbsp dry white wine
3 tbsp white wine vinegar
4 ice cubes
Juice of ½ lemon (optional)
Salt and cayenne pepper to taste
1 tbsp whole fresh tarragon leaves

1 Finely chop the shallots, crush the white peppercorns and whisk the egg yolks. Melt the butter in a pan and set aside to cool.

2 Place the shallots, peppercorns, chopped tarragon, wine and vinegar in a separate pan. Cook until the mixture reduces to around 2 tbsp.

3 Strain the reduction into a bowl set above a pan of simmering water. Whisk in the egg yolk until the mixture begins to thicken. Add ice cubes to the pan to cool the water.

4 Drizzle in the melted butter. Add a little lemon juice if desired and salt and pepper to taste. Whisk thoroughly.

5 Remove from the heat. Stir in the whole tarragon leaves. Serve warm.

Other uses
❧ Pile up tarragon, basil, parsley and radishes to make the Persian side dish *sabzi khordan*.
❧ Add bittersweet tarragon-infused white wine vinegar or *fines herbes* (see page 29) to bakes, roasts or salads.

STYLE
TARKHUN (TARRAGON-ADE)

The tarragon-flavoured Georgian soft drink *tarkhun* was invented at the end of the nineteenth century, in the quest for a natural syrup for lemonade. Add traditional bright green natural colouring to create a fun drink for kids' parties.

Serves 6
For the tarragon syrup:
225g (1 cup) sugar
¹/₈ tsp bicarbonate of soda
Large handful of tarragon leaves
3 ice cubes
Juice of 1 large lemon (2–3 tbsp)

For the tarkhun:
2–4 tbsp tarragon syrup (see above)
1 litre (1 quart) sparkling water
4 drops natural green food colouring (optional)
12 ice cubes

1 Mix the sugar and 85ml (1/3 cup) of water in a pan. Bring to a boil, stirring continuously. Add the bicarbonate of soda and tarragon leaves and cook for 1 minute.

2 Let the syrup cool slightly. Blitz until smooth in a blender. Add the three ice cubes and the lemon juice. Blend again.

3 Strain through a fine mesh sieve. Place in the fridge to cool.

4 Mix the tarragon syrup with the sparkling water to make basic *tarkhun*. Add a few drops of green food colouring (if desired) and ice cubes to chill.

Other uses
❧ Create the Slovenian festive dessert *potica* by rolling ground walnuts, tarragon, quark (soft cheese), hazelnuts and pumpkin seeds into leavened dough.
❧ Muddle greeny-grey tarragon into a pink, gin fizz cocktail with soda, elderflower liqueur and grapefruit juice.

BORAGE
Borago officinalis, Boraginaceae family

Borage's cheerful blue, star-shaped flowers characterise a herb with joyful associations throughout herbal history. Hairy leaves and stems link it to other Boraginaceae family species such as forget-me-not (*Myosotis*), green alkanet (*Pentaglottis sempervirens*) and comfrey (*Symphytum*). A traditional and lovely addition to the kitchen garden for its hint-of-cucumber-tasting flowers and leaves, and the beauty of its blooms, borage also works its magic as a balancing and stress-busting medicinal herb, most typically under the guise of starflower oil.

❧ THE DESCRIPTION Borage's five-petalled blue flowers are its most identifiable feature 'distinguished from those of every plant in this order by their prominent black anthers, which form a cone in the centre and have been described as their beauty spot.' (Mrs M. Grieve, *A Modern Herbal*, 1931). The whole plant is rough and hairy with tall, round, hollow stems and large, oval and pointed, deep green, alternate leaves.

❧ THE NAME No one seems to know exactly where the word *borage* comes from. One theory suggests the Latin *corage*, combining *cor* meaning 'heart' and *ago* 'I bring'; another gives 'bugloss', a common synonym for borage and other Boraginaceae family species. This derives from the Ancient Greek *buglosson* meaning 'ox's tongue', pointing to borage's hairy, tongue-shaped leaves. *Officinalis* refers to a medicinal plant.

❧ THE PLACE Although Mrs M. Grieve traces the origins of *Borago officinalis* to Aleppo in Syria, it is more likely to hail from North Africa. It is now widely cultivated and naturalised throughout much of the temperate world, including Europe and North and South America, where it 'flourishes in ordinary soil' (*A Modern Herbal*, 1931) in gardens and the wild. To grow, choose reasonably light well-drained soil, preferably in sun.

❧ THE TIME Cultivate borage from division of rootstocks in spring, by cuttings in summer and autumn, or sow seeds from mid-spring to early summer or in autumn. It also happily self-seeds. 'Borage floures and flourishes most part of all Summer, and till Autumne be far spent', records John Gerard (*Herball*, 1597). Mrs M. Grieve suggests gathering leaves 'on a fine day', when the 'plant is coming into flower'.

❧ THE VIRTUES 'Syrup made of the floures of Borrage comforteth the heart, purgeth melancholy, and quieteth the phrenticke or lunaticke person', notes John Gerard. Borage seed oil – or starflower oil – is now known to contain high levels of Gamma-linolenic acid (GLA), used to benefit skin, treat arthritis and prevent inflammation. A few young leaves are also great in salads, while the flowers make the prettiest garnish.

Plate 36

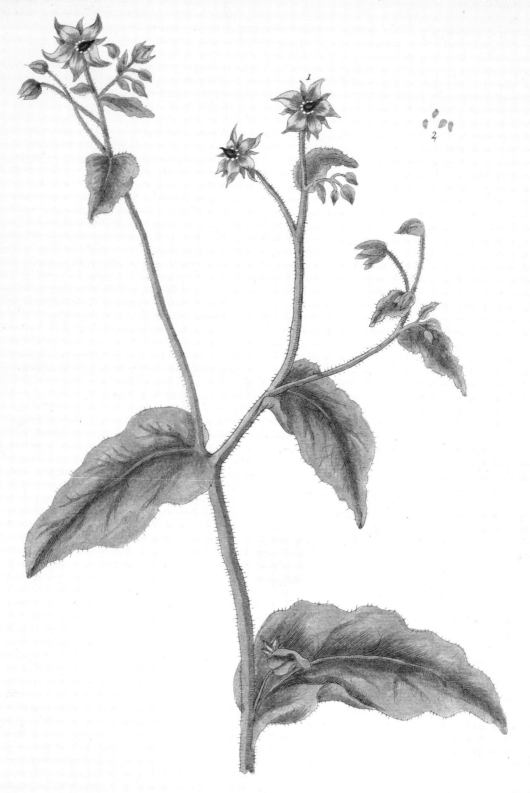

Borrage ⎰ 1 Flower ⎱ Borago
⎱ 2 Seed ⎰

Eliz. Blackwell delin. sculp et Pinx.

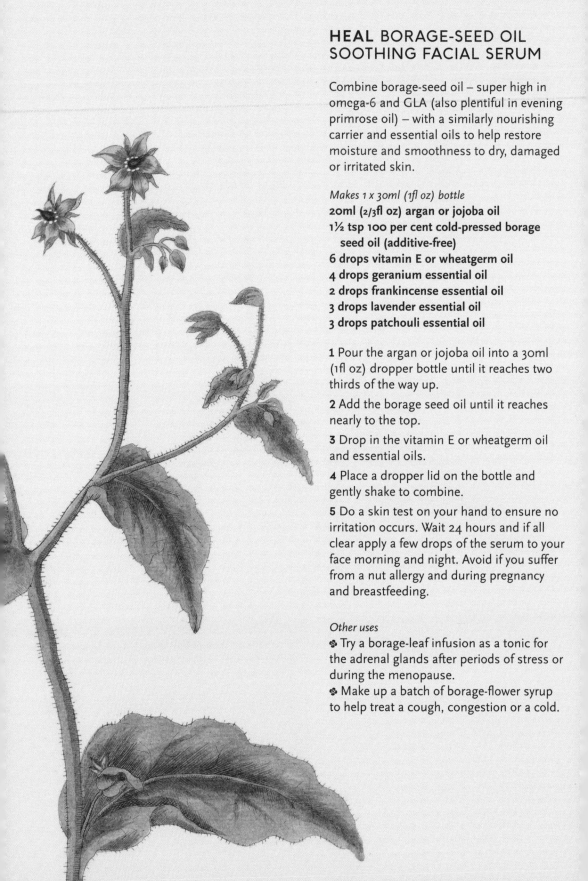

HEAL BORAGE-SEED OIL SOOTHING FACIAL SERUM

Combine borage-seed oil – super high in omega-6 and GLA (also plentiful in evening primrose oil) – with a similarly nourishing carrier and essential oils to help restore moisture and smoothness to dry, damaged or irritated skin.

Makes 1 x 30ml (1fl oz) bottle
20ml (2/3fl oz) argan or jojoba oil
1½ tsp 100 per cent cold-pressed borage seed oil (additive-free)
6 drops vitamin E or wheatgerm oil
4 drops geranium essential oil
2 drops frankincense essential oil
3 drops lavender essential oil
3 drops patchouli essential oil

1 Pour the argan or jojoba oil into a 30ml (1fl oz) dropper bottle until it reaches two thirds of the way up.

2 Add the borage seed oil until it reaches nearly to the top.

3 Drop in the vitamin E or wheatgerm oil and essential oils.

4 Place a dropper lid on the bottle and gently shake to combine.

5 Do a skin test on your hand to ensure no irritation occurs. Wait 24 hours and if all clear apply a few drops of the serum to your face morning and night. Avoid if you suffer from a nut allergy and during pregnancy and breastfeeding.

Other uses
❧ Try a borage-leaf infusion as a tonic for the adrenal glands after periods of stress or during the menopause.
❧ Make up a batch of borage-flower syrup to help treat a cough, congestion or a cold.

NOURISH
BORAGE-LEAF RAVIOLI

Pick early spring, tender borage leaves to add to the delicious cheese and herb filling of this traditional western Ligurian ravioli.

Makes 16 ravioli
450g (1lb) tender borage leaves
250g (1 cup) ricotta cheese
100g (1 cup) grated Parmesan, plus extra to serve
A grating of fresh nutmeg
300g (2½ cups) plain flour, plus extra for dusting
3 eggs
16 fresh sage leaves
60g (¼ cup) butter
Sea salt to taste

1 Clean the borage leaves, remove the stalks and simmer in boiling water until tender. Drain well and finely chop. Place in a bowl.

2 Add the ricotta and Parmesan, nutmeg and a pinch of sea salt. Mix well and shape into 16 balls.

3 Place a volcano-shaped heap of the flour on a clean surface. Make a well in the top, crack in the eggs and mix and knead to form a dough. Shape into a ball, cover with a cloth and leave to rest for 20 minutes.

4 Flour a clean surface, roll out the dough and cut 16 circles using a 12cm (5in) cutter. Place a ball of stuffing onto one half of each circle and fold into a half-moon. Pinch the edges between your fingertips to seal.

5 Cook the ravioli in salted boiling water for 3–4 minutes, then draine. Fry the sage leaves in the butter.

6 Spoon hot sage butter over the ravioli and garnish with Parmesan. Eat in moderation.

Other uses
❀ Dip tender leaves in batter and fry until crisp to make Roman-style borage fritters.
❀ Make a vivid green cold soup of blended cucumber, almonds and borage leaves.

STYLE
STARFLOWER PIMM'S

The quintessential, British summer cocktail, Pimm's is even more attractive with a garnish of fresh blue borage flowers alongside the usual sliced fruit. Add a further touch of glamour by swapping lemonade for Champagne and serving in flute glasses as a Pimm's Royale.

Makes 1 x 1 litre (1 quart) jug
200ml (8fl oz) Pimm's No. 1
600ml (24fl oz) lemonade
4 thin slices of cucumber
4 strawberries, hulled and quartered
4 thin slices of orange
4 mint leaves, washed
At least 12 borage flowers
Plenty of ice

1 Half-fill a 1 litre (1 quart) jug with ice. Pour in the Pimms, then the lemonade.

2 Add the cucumber, strawberries and orange. Tear in a handful of mint leaves. Stir gently and add ice.

3 Pour the Pimm's into four highball glasses and garnish with at least 3 borage flowers each.

Other uses
❀ Plant bee- and butterfly-attracting borage plants next to tomatoes, squash or strawberries to help increase yield.
❀ Freeze borage flowers in ice cubes or ice lollies for the sweetest summer drinks or cooling treats.

CALENDULA
Calendula officinalis, Asteraceae family

Sunny-flowered calendula, known as pot or common marigold adds a welcome burst of uplifting colour to the garden right through late spring, summer, autumn and 'sometimes in winter, if it be mild' (Nicholas Culpeper, *Complete Herbal*, 1653). Calendula also has myriad uses – as an edible flower and aromatic leaf, a skin-soothing essential oil and a saffron-like food colouring or dye. No surprise then that the cultivation of this popular and cherished 'pot' herb has continued for millennia from the days of ancient Egypt, Greece, Rome, Persia and India to modern times.

❀ THE DESCRIPTION 'The common marigold is familiar to everyone, with its pale green leaves and golden orange flowers', notes Mrs M. Grieve in *A Modern Herbal* (1931). Not to be confused with the smaller-flowered French or African marigold (*Tagetes*), calendula has yellow or orange daisy-like flowers with a double row of petals and 'broad, thicke and rough leaves of an overworn green colour, not unlike those of Plantaine' (John Gerard, *Herball*, 1597).

❀ THE NAME Calendula's common and genus name meaning 'little calendar' stems from the Latin *Calends* (*Kalendae*). This could refer to calendula's regular clock-like action of opening and closing with the sun. Also historically known as 'chrysanthemum, 'marigold', or '*Caltha*', the species name *Calendula officinalis* was eventually made official by Carl Linnaeus in 1753. *Officinalis* points to calendula's medicinal benefits.

❀ THE PLACE 'The Marigold is a native of south Europe, but perfectly hardy in this country [United Kingdom], and easy to grow', writes Mrs M. Grieve. Now thought to be native to Europe, Asia and Africa, calendula has also been widely introduced to temperate regions of the globe. It prefers light, poor, free-draining soil in full sun and flourishes in both garden borders or containers.

❀ THE TIME Sow seeds in situ in late spring for flowers within two months, or in autumn for bushier plants and plentiful flowers the following year. 'They require no other cultivation but to keep them clean from weeds and to thin out where too close', advises Mrs M. Grieve. She also suggests drying flowers immediately after collection to maintain colour, by placing on sheets of paper and leaving in a warm place.

❀ THE VIRTUES Fresh or dried calendula flowers were 'much used in potlets, broths and drinks, being comfortable to the heart and spirits', observed Nicholas Culpeper. They were also used to soothe the 'hot swellings' of smallpox and measles. Today, calendula's anti-inflammatory and antiviral properties are widely harnessed in skin treatments, while the vitamin-rich leaves and bittersweet flowers work well in salads.

Plate 106.

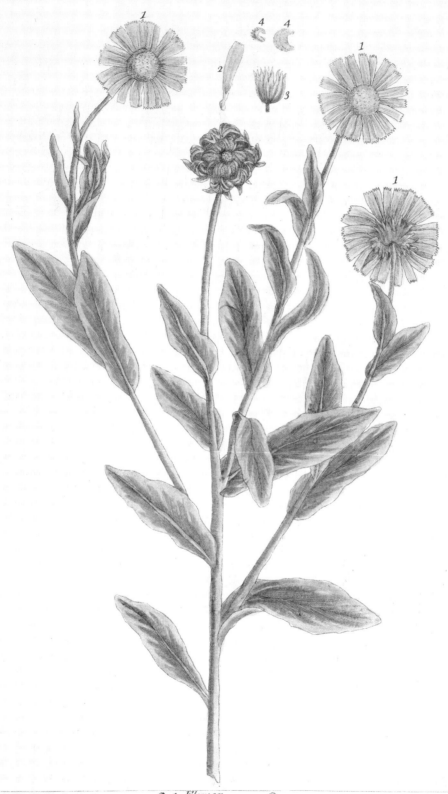

Mary golds.

iz. Blackwell delin. sculp. et Pinx.

1. Flower
2. Flower separate
3. Calix
4. Seed

Calendula.

HEAL SKIN-SOOTHING BATH SOAK

Combine the healing power of calendula flowers – used for centuries as a traditional first-aid remedy – with similarly soothing oatmeal, Epsom salts and lavender for a restorative and skin-calming bath soak. Harvest calendula flowers (in fine weather) and lavender buds (before full bloom) and dry in a warm place – or source pre-dried flowers from a store.

Makes 2 x 500g (17½fl oz) jars
175g (2 cups) organic oats
200g (1 cup) Epsom salts
2 tbsp bicarbonate of soda
2 tbsp dried lavender flowers
4 tbsp dried calendula flowers
5–10 drops lavender essential oil
Muslin sachet bags

1 Gently grind the oats using a pestle and mortar, or whizz slowly in a blender. Ensure some texture remains. Place in a bowl.

2 Add the Epsom salts, bicarbonate of soda, flowers, and essential oil.

3 Stir gently until combined. Pour into two 500ml (17½fl oz) airtight sterilised glass lidded jars.

4 To use, spoon some mixture into a muslin sachet bag. Secure by tying the ends, then place the bag in the bathtub to infuse. The sachet can also be used to wash, massage and exfoliate the skin.

Other uses
❧ Prepare a batch of calendula-infused oil as the base for calendula soap, body butter, lotion bars, lip balm or salad dressing.
❧ Use calendula-infused tea as a sore-throat gargle, digestive, face wash or to help regulate the menstrual cycle.

NOURISH RAINBOW FLOWER SUMMER ROLLS

Add calendula's glowing orange petals to a fresh summer roll of aromatic herbs, crunchy vegetables, bean sprouts and noodles.

Makes 12 rolls
½ cucumber
1 carrot, peeled
4 garden radishes
2 spring onions
150g (1½ cups) bean sprouts
½ tbsp rice vinegar
½ tbsp granulated sugar
1 tsp soy sauce
Juice of ½ lime
100g (3½oz) rice vermicelli noodles
½ tsp sesame oil
12 round rice-paper wrappers (around 20cm/8in diameter)
Mixed small bunch of Thai basil, coriander and mint
2 tbsp fresh calendula petals, washed
Peanut or soy dipping sauce, to serve

1 Finely slice the cucumber, carrot, radishes and spring onions. Cook the bean sprouts for 1–2 minutes and drain.

2 Whisk the vinegar, sugar, soy sauce and lime juice in a large bowl. Add the chopped vegetables and bean sprouts and toss.

3 Break up the noodles and cook as per the pack instructions. Coat in the sesame oil in a bowl.

4 Soak the rice-paper wrappers for a few seconds in cool water to soften. Fill each one with torn basil, mint and coriander leaves, and calendula petals followed by equal parts vegetable mixture and noodles. Fold in the ends and roll. Repeat until all the mix is used.

Other uses
❧ Fresh calendula petals, goat's cheese and rocket is a great salad mix or pizza topping.
❧ Make natural orange food colouring by steeping dried calendula petals in boiled water.

STYLE
CALENDULA SUNRISE SOAP

Calendula's skin-soothing properties and pretty orange petals, plus uplifting sweet orange essential oil, make a lovely child-friendly soap. Source a soap base that's free from sodium lauryl sulphate (SLS) and palm oil.

Makes 6 small bars
450g (1lb) vegetable-based (shea butter, argan oil or oatmeal) melt-and-pour soap
1 tsp shea butter
1½ tbsp calendula-infused sweet almond oil (see pages 18–19)
10 drops sweet orange essential oil
½ cup dried calendula flower petals (removed from flower heads)
Rubbing alcohol in a spray bottle
Silicon soap mould (6 small cavities)

1 Place the soap mould on a solid surface such as a chopping board.

2 Cut the soap base into cubes and place in a bowl. Add the shea butter. Heat over a pan of boiling water until melted. Remove from the heat.

3 Stir in the sweet almond oil, sweet orange essential oil and calendula flower petals. Then divide the mixture evenly between the cavities in the mould. Wipe away any spillages before the soap sets.

4 Immediately spray the top of each surface with a little rubbing alcohol to minimise bubbles.

5 Allow the soap to set for 1–2 hours at room temperature. Remove from the mould, wrap in wax paper and use or gift as desired.

Other uses
❧ Give cocktails an earthy blush with a simple syrup (see page 19) of calendula flowers, honey and water.
❧ Grow eye-catching *Calendula officinalis* cultivars such as the ruffled 'Pink Surprise', 'Neon' with double blooms, or black-centered 'Golden Princess' for a dazzling display.

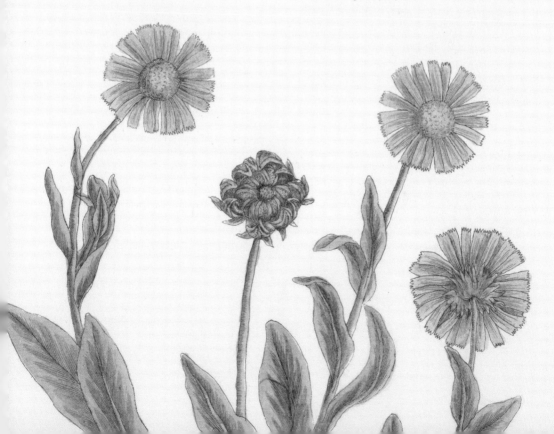

CORNFLOWER
Centaurea cyanus, Asteraceae family

Once a common sight of the cornfield, meadow and hedgerow, the cornflower is of such a beautiful and arresting blue hue (in its most recognisable form) that it even inspired the name of a colour. Now rarely seen growing wild in the wheat, barley, rye or oat fields of its native Europe, this lovely wildflower thankfully survives and flourishes in gardens, parks and along verges. It has been cultivated over the centuries for its ornamental charm, as an edible flower and natural colourant, and as an eye-soothing medicinal herb.

❀ THE DESCRIPTION Mrs M. Grieve (*A Modern Herbal*, 1931) describes cornflower as having wiry, angular stems and narrow, long, alternate leaves covered in cobwebby down. The 'flowers grow solitary, and of necessity upon long stalks to raise them among the corn' with scaly bracts from which flowers emerge, the inner florets being 'a pale purplish rose colour', the 'bright blue ray florets' widely spread and 'cut into'.

❀ THE NAME Blue bottle and bachelor's buttons are two of the cornflower's common names, the latter referring to the young men who wore the flower in their buttonholes to declare love. The botanical name *Centaurea cyanus* is steeped in mythology – *Centaurea* after the ancient Greek Centaur Chiron who 'taught mankind the healing virtue of herbs'; *cyanus* after Cyanus, a youthful devotee of the Roman goddess Flora, who loved cornflowers most of all, or the Greek word *kyanos*, meaning 'dark blue'.

❀ THE PLACE Before the widespread use of herbicides, whole fields studded with cornflowers were a common sight, possibly as far back as Neolithic times. Today, it's more usual to find them cropping up in planned wildflower meadows, cottage gardens and informal borders. Grow in beds or good-sized pots in well-drained soil in full sun, perhaps alongside contrasting red poppies or orange calendulas (page 38) or as a pollinator-attracting companion plant.

❀ THE TIME 'Transplant cornflowers in your garden especially toward the full of the moon', suggests Nicholas Culpeper (*Complete Herbal*, 1653), and 'they will grow more double than they are, and many times change their colour'. For an early summer bloom, sow seeds where they are to flower in early spring, or in autumn for summer colour next year. Harvest flowers when the centre petals are not completely open.

❀ THE VIRTUES The powdered or dried leaves of cornflowers were historically used to treat bruises and broken veins, while 'the juice dropped in the eyes taketh away the heat and inflammation in them' (*Complete Herbal*, 1653). It is now known that cornflowers contain high levels of flavonoids called anthocyanins, which have strong antioxidant and anti-inflammatory properties as well as delivering that fabulous blue.

Plate 270.

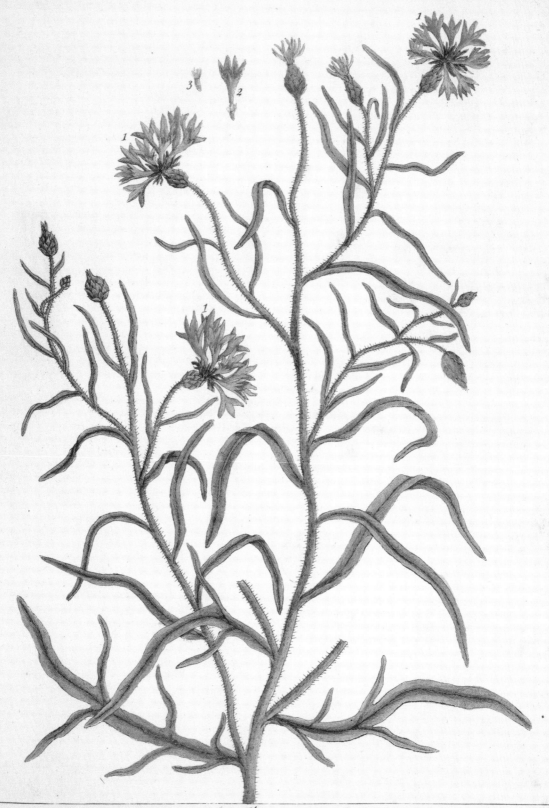

Small Blue-Bottle.

Eliz. Blackwell delin. sculp. et Pinx.

1. Flower.
2. Flower separate.
3. Seed.

Cyanus minor.

HEAL
SOOTHING MISTER

Cornflower hydrosol – steam-distilled flower water with traces of the essential oil within (see page 116) – is traditionally renowned for its therapeutic properties. Spritz onto muslin squares and place over swollen eyes, mist directly onto face to help tone oily skin, or diffuse into the air to help restore calm – perfect for travelling.

Makes 1 x 120ml (4fl oz) mister
**120ml (4fl oz) cornflower hydrosol
(homemade – see page 116 – or
store bought)
120ml (4fl oz) blue glass mister bottle**

1 Prepare a cornflower hydrosol according to the instructions for Rose Hydrosol (see page 116), substituting fresh or dried cornflower petals for rose petals. Or source a premade cornflower hydrosol from a store.

2 Decant the cornflower hydrosol into a 120ml (4fl oz) bottle – choose cobalt blue glass to protect ingredients from UV rays and reference the beautiful blue cornflower ingredient inside.

3 Seal with a spray cap and mist around face, body or home as required.

Other uses
❧ Cornflower tea made from an infusion of fresh or dried petals is thought to ease mild constipation.
❧ Spritz body with cornflower hydrosol before applying massage oil to help promote feelings of peace.

NOURISH
EARL BLUE TEA

Add to Earl Grey tea's aromatic, sensual, bergamot flavour with a peppering of uplifting blue cornflower petals. Brew in a glass teapot for one, for an extra layer of indulgence and to watch the pretty tea infuse.

Makes 1 x 135ml (5fl oz) jar
**125g (4½oz) loose-leaf Earl Grey tea
10g (1/3oz) dried cornflower petals
Slices of lemon, to serve**

1 Dry cornflowers by hanging flower stems in loose bunches (see pages 16–17) then removing petals by hand; or source from a store.

2 Combine loose-leaf Earl Grey tea and the dried petals in a bowl. Mix well and decant into a 135g (5fl oz) airtight jar.

3 To brew the perfect cup of Earl Blue tea, heat water in a kettle to almost boiling. Swirl a little of this water in a 1-cup (250ml) glass teapot to warm it up. Discard the water. Add 2 tsp of Earl Blue Tea and leave to brew for 3 minutes. Serve black with a slice of lemon and a cornflower-petal topped cupcake.

Other uses
❧ Add slightly spicy-tasting cornflower petals to salads, soups and sweet or savoury treats.
❧ Grind dried cornflower petals in a pestle and mortar to make natural food colouring – play around with pink, mauve or white cultivars to create different shades.

STYLE
CORNFLOWER BATH BOMB

Celebrate the beauty of cornflower blue, a favourite colour of Dutch painter Johannes Vermeer (1632–1675), by adding cornflower petals to a skin-soothing, lavender-scented bath bomb.

Makes 6 x 5cm (2in) diameter bath bombs
300g (1½ cups) bicarbonate of soda
100g (1/3 cup) citric acid
100g (½ cup) Epsom salts
1 tbsp sweet almond oil or melted shea butter (optional)
20 drops lavender essential oil
4 tbsp witch hazel (in a spray bottle)
Small handful of dried cornflower petals
6 spherical (50mm/2in) two-part bath bomb moulds

1 Combine the bicarbonate of soda, citric acid and Epsom salts in a large bowl. Add sweet almond oil or melted shea butter, if desired.

2 Add the lavender essential oil, stirring continuously. Spritz with enough witch hazel until the mixture is just firm enough to form a ball. Too much liquid will cause the mixture to start fizzing.

3 Place a few cornflower petals in the bottom half of each mould. Then fill both halves of each mould with bath-bomb mixture just higher than the top. Press the halves together to make spheres.

4 Remove the top half of each mould and tap gently to ease it off. Leave for 30 minutes to set.

5 Remove the remaining half-mould and place the bomb on a clean surface for 24 hours until fully dry.

6 Keep in an airtight container. Dissolve in a warm bath and soak in the cornflower lavender goodness.

Other uses
❀ Combine cornflowers, bearded wheat, Helichrysum or strawflower (*Xerochrysum bracteatum* syn. *Helichrysum bracteatum*) and baby's breath (*Gypsophila paniculata*) in a dried flower garland or bouquet.
❀ Create a pollinator-friendly wildflower mini-meadow with blue cornflowers, red poppies and white ox-eye daisies.

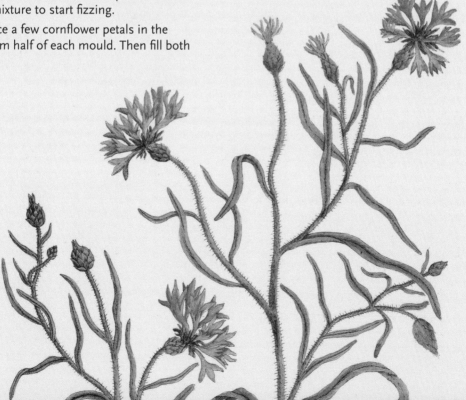

CHAMOMILE
Chamaemelum nobile, Asteraceae family

The daisy-like, apple-scented, unassuming yet much-cherished blooms of chamomile have traditionally been used to 'comforteth', 'easeth' and 'dissolveth' a range of ailments from digestive issues, malaria-like fevers and joint pain to general 'weariness' (Nicholas Culpeper, *Complete Herbal*, 1653). While *Chamaemelum nobile* (Roman or true chamomile) is the *Camomile* and *Cammomil* spoken of by Culpeper and John Gerard (*Herball*, 1597), its close relative *Matricaria chamomilla* (German or false chamomile) has long been cultivated for its healing powers too.

❧ **THE DESCRIPTION** Creeping perennial chamomile has free-branching stems, and 'leaves which are divided into thread-like segments, the fineness of which gives the whole plant a feathery appearance' (Mrs M. Grieve, *A Modern Herbal*, 1931). Single flowers with white petals and a yellow conical centre (less raised than non-perennial German chamomile) are sweet scented, as are the leaves and stems.

❧ **THE NAME** Although the species name *Chamaemelum nobile*, published in 1785, replaced Carl Linnaeus's *Anthemis nobilis*, Mrs M. Grieve was still using the latter in 1931. *Chamaemelum* stems from the ancient Greek *khamaimelon* from *khamai* meaning 'on the ground' and *melon* for 'apple', alluding to chamomile's distinctive apple aroma and taste. *Nobile* refers to this historical plant's status as a 'well-known' or 'knowable' herb.

❧ **THE PLACE** This native of the United Kingdom, France, Spain and Portugal is now naturalised throughout central Europe. It grows on any light, well-drained soil in full sun and is best cut back after flowering to keep the plant compact. Known as the 'plant's physician' for its seeming ability to cure nearby ailing plants, chamomile also attracts beneficial pollinators to borders or pots. For a chamomile lawn choose the non-flowering cultivar 'Treneague'.

❧ **THE TIME** Mrs M. Grieve suggests sowing chamomile in late spring or early summer by seed, transplanting to 'permanent quarters' outside when large enough. 'Treneague', the lawn chamomile, can be propagated only from cuttings taken in autumn. Harvest chamomile flowerheads in the late morning, throughout the summer blooming period, when they are at their fullest.

❧ **THE VIRTUES** Cure-all chamomile was traditionally 'esteem'd good' for the stomach, colic, jaundice, kidney stones, urinary problems, fever, inflammation and tumors (Elizabeth Blackwell, *A Curious Herbal*, 1737–39). Today, it is mainly used in the form of a calming tea for mild anxiety or insomnia. Roman chamomile essential oil, which is blue, is anti-inflammatory and traditionally used for eczema.

Plate 298.

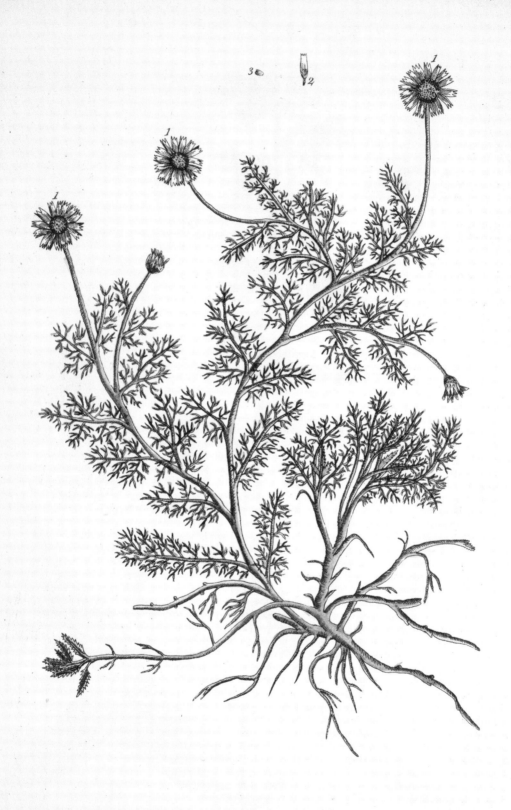

..bz: Blackwell delin. sculp. et Pinx.

Camomile.

1. *Flower.*
2. *Flower separate.*
3. *Seed.*

Chamaemelum.

HEAL SOOTHE-ME CHAMOMILE TEA

Chamomile tea was used in ancient Egypt to treat fevers, and in Rome for skin-soothing preparations and fragrance as well as a beverage. Today, its applications include a cooling eye treatment and a skin or hair rinse, as well as a sedative and relaxing bedtime brew.

Makes 10 teabags
20g (2/3oz) dried chamomile flowers
10 x small unbleached paper teabags
Small card tags

1 Fill each paper teabag with around 1 tbsp of dried chamomile flowers.

2 Pull the drawstrings to close and label as chamomile tea using a small card tag.

3 To prepare the tea, steep 1 bag in a cup of just-boiled water for 3–5 minutes. Drink hot

to benefit from a calming, digestive brew. Use the cooled teabag as a restorative compress for eyes or skin.

Other uses
❧ Place a few drops of Roman chamomile essential oil onto a handkerchief or muslin cloth and inhale to help combat stress or insomnia.
❧ Use a few drops of Roman chamomile essential oil in a face lotion or shampoo to help soothe irritated skin or scalp.

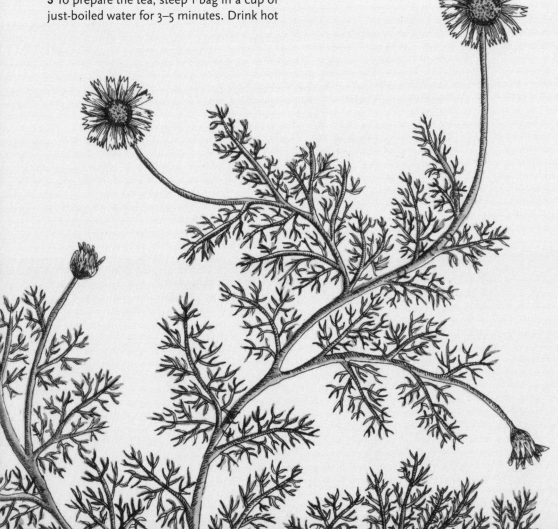

NOURISH
EARTH-APPLE PORRIDGE

The dainty apple scent and nourishing actions of chamomile flowers are deliciously nutritious in a bowl of porridge, overnight soaked oats or granola. Experiment with ingredients until you get your perfect blend.

Serves 2
90g (1 cup) rolled oats
250ml (1 cup) chamomile tea (see opposite)
Handful of dried chamomile flowers
Handful of flaked almonds
30g (1oz) knob of butter
250ml (1 cup) almond milk
¼ tsp salt
2 tbsp almond butter
Honey or maple syrup to drizzle

1 Place the oats in a medium pan, cover with chamomile tea and soak for 10 minutes.

2 Sauté the flowers, then the almonds, in a knob of butter for 1 minute.

3 Pour the milk over the soaked oats. Bring to a boil, add the salt and simmer gently for 3–5 minutes, stirring frequently. Remove from the heat and allow to stand for 1 minute.

4 Divide the porridge into two bowls, swirling a tbsp of almond butter into each one.

5 Garnish with the sautéed flowers and almonds, drizzle with honey or maple syrup, and serve while hot.

Other uses
❧ Make chamomile cordial to dilute with sparkling water or drizzle over ice cream.
❧ Add pretty white and yellow fresh chamomile blooms to a green salad.

STYLE
CHAMOMILE LAWN

Dispense with the regular mowing, fertilising and edging of a lawn in favour of a fragrant, springy chamomile alternative that releases a calming apple-like scent with every footstep. For a low-growing, pollen-free option, go for the mat-forming *Chamaemelum nobile* 'Treneague', available as plants or turf – also a favourite filler plant for Elizabethan knot gardens.

Covers 1 sq m (10 sq ft)
100 x *Chamomile nobile* 'Treneague' plug plants or 1 sq m (10 sq ft) of turf

1 Choose a sunny spot suitable for a lawn and remove stones and all traces of perennial weeds. Level and dig in grit to improve drainage if your soil is heavy.

2 Space plants 10–20cm (4–8in) apart, or unroll chamomile lawn turf and lay. Water well.

3 Abstain from walking on your lawn for at least 12 weeks and avoid heavy use during the first year. A good way around this is to make a footpath through the centre of the lawn.

4 Enjoy your chamomile lawn's zingy colour and scent, digging out any weeds as they appear.

Other uses
❧ Infuse vodka with dried chamomile flowers, honey and lemon zest for a floral, grassy chamomile liqueur.
❧ A daisy-chain of chamomile flowers worn as a midsummer necklace or hair garland is the pagan way to attract a lover.

CHICORY
Cichorium intybus, Asteraceae family

Formerly known as *succorie* or *succory*, common or garden chicory bears some resemblance to a sky-blue-flowered dandelion. Historically, the herb was grown for its bitter leaves, medicinal properties, potential as a fodder crop, and its long, sweet taproot from which the natural sweetener inulin and chicory coffee substitute are derived. Cultivars include red chicory, known as radicchio, which Pliny refers to as a salad vegetable, and the familiar witloof or Belgian chicory that is 'forced' (deprived of light) to produce white, less bitter leaves. *Cichorium endivia* or true endive is also a close cousin.

❧ **THE DESCRIPTION** Plate 177 (opposite) of Elizabeth Blackwell's *A Curious Herbal* (1737–39) depicts '*Cichorium Sativum*' now known as *Cichorium intybus* var. *sativum*, cultivated for its root. Plate 183 of her book shows 'Wild Succory' or '*Cichorium sylvestre*' – *Cichorium intybus* in a yet wilder form. Both have long, narrower leaves than true endive, 'more cut in and torn at the edges' (Nicholas Culpeper, *Complete Herbal*, 1653).

❧ **THE NAME** The species names *intybus* (wild or garden chicory) and *endivia* (true endive) were given by Carl Linnaeus in *Species Plantarum* (1753), probably from the Greek name *entybon*. *Cichorium* is thought to stem from the ancient Greek *kikhórion* meaning 'field' or 'endive', while *intybus* stems from the Greek for 'to cut', referring to chicory's toothed leaves, or the Latin *tubus* on account of its hollow stem.

❧ **THE PLACE** Native to Europe and parts of Asia, *Cichorium intybus* has been cultivated since at least 300 BC. It is now widely naturalised in parts of North America, Australia and China, often found growing wild along roadsides. To grow *Cichorium intybus*, provide a sunny spot and fertile, well-drained soil. It's also possible to grow radicchio and to force your own Belgian chicory.

❧ **THE TIME** Propagate from seed sown under cover in autumn or spring. Harvest leaves in summer and roots from autumn to spring. To blanch or force the leaves, Mrs M. Grieve (*A Modern Herbal*, 1931) suggests digging up plants in autumn, cutting off the leaves, and exposing roots to the air for two weeks before planting them in deep boxes of sand or light soil.

❧ **THE VIRTUES** A decoction of chicory made with wine is 'very effectual against long lingering agues', writes Nicholas Culpeper (an 'ague' being a feverish illness). He also prescribes it for jaundice, passions of the heart and inflamed eyes. Today, chicory is mainly prized for the high levels of the sweet-tasting fibre inulin found in its root, which can help with digestive issues and makes chicory beverages palatable.

Plate 177

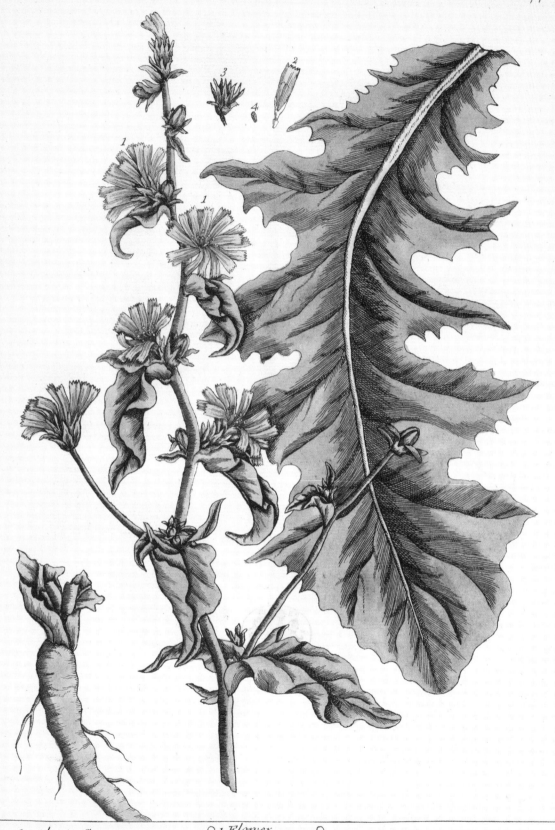

Garden Succory

Eliz. Blackwell delin sculp. et Pinx.

1. Flower.
2. Flower separate.
3. Calix.
4. Seed.

Cichorium sativum or Seris.

HEAL
CHICORY COFFEE

This increasingly popular coffee substitute, originating in nineteenth-century France and still a traditional beverage in the cafés of New Orleans, is made from dehydrated and ground chicory root. Not only is it caffeine free, it also contains the sweet gut-friendly fibre inulin.

Makes 1 x 500ml (17½fl oz) jar

Large bunch (8–10) fresh chicory roots
Almond or hemp milk, to serve (optional)
Coffee grinder

1 Harvest chicory roots between autumn and spring when at their most nutritious. Wash away soil, blot with kitchen towel and leave in a warm place to dry.

2 Cut the roots into 2.5cm (1in) pieces, lay out on a baking sheet and dehydrate in an oven at around 80°C (180°F) or the lowest setting until golden brown. You could also use a dehydrator. Allow to cool completely.

3 Grind into coarse grains using a coffee or spice grinder. Store in an airtight 500ml (17½fl oz) jar.

4 Brew as you would coffee, using around 2 tps of chicory grains for every 250ml (1 cup) just-boiled water. Add a dash of almond or hemp milk for a creamier concoction.

Other uses
❧ Drink a mild decoction of chicory root to help support the liver and gallbladder.
❧ Simmer chicory root with water and coconut sugar to make a syrup (see page 19) and use as a natural sweetener in coffee or baking.

NOURISH
FAVE E CICORIA

This traditional recipe of mashed fava beans and sautéed chicory leaves hails from Puglia, Italy, where it was traditionally made in earthenware jars by a fire and eaten on its own, or with bread or potatoes. Chicory leaves are not widely available in stores, so grow or forage (with a guide).

Serves 2

250g (8oz) dried fava beans (shelled)
Large bunch of 'wild' chicory (*Cichorium intybus*) leaves
3 tbsp extra virgin olive oil, plus extra to serve
2 garlic cloves
Sea salt and black pepper to taste

1 Soak the beans overnight for at least 12 hours. Strain and pour into a pan.

2 Cover with 750ml (3 cups) of water and cook for around 40 minutes until soft and falling apart. Puree with a hand blender. Stir in 1 tbsp of extra virgin olive oil. Add sea salt to taste.

3 Wash the chicory leaves and cut off the hard stems. Blanch in boiling water for 3 minutes, then drain.

4 Chop the garlic and sauté it in the remaining oil until golden. Remove the garlic and sauté the leaves in the garlic-infused oil until tender. Add sea salt and black pepper to taste.

5 Spoon the bean mash into bowls, add a swirl of olive oil, top with the sautéed leaves and eat immediately.

Other uses
❧ Blanch and toss tender chicory leaves in a salad. Pick in spring or autumn as summer heat can make the leaves taste bitter.
❧ Pickle chicory flower buds, like capers, in white wine vinegar, honey and salt with a little ground ginger, cinnamon or coriander.

STYLE
CHICORY O'CLOCK

Introduced by Swedish botanist Carl Linnaeus in his *Philosophia Botanica* (1751), a floral clock aims to tell the time using the opening and closing times of flowers – a lovely way to introduce children to plants and flowers. It's not known if Linnaeus ever planted his '*Horologium Florae*' but his specimen list did include chicory among other herbs.

Makes 1 flower clock patch

Chicory (*Cichorium intybus*), Icelandic poppy (*Papaver nudicaule*) and calendula (*Calendula officinalis*) seeds/seedlings
Add complementary 'flower clock' plants such as tulip (*Tulipa*), crocus (*Crocus sativus*), daisy (*Bellis perennis*) and Californian poppy (*Eschscholzia californica*)

1 Mark out a patch of herb garden or border for 'flower clock' specimens. Sow seeds or plant up seedlings according to the instructions on the pack or pot.

2 Wait until flowers bloom and then note the time when they open and close. Chicory blooms from July to September in its second year (from seed), with flowers opening in the early morning and closing around 5 hours later. Icelandic poppy blooms from May to August in its second year (from seed), with flowers opening during sunlight but closing at night or on a dull day. Calendula blooms from June to September in its first year (from seed), with flowers opening at sunrise and closing at sunset.

Other uses

❖ Make a blue dye from chicory leaves or a yellow-brown one from the blue flowers (see nettle, page 153 for dyeing processes and ideas).
❖ Crystallise chicory's gorgeous sky blue flowers (see page 117) to make lovely garnishes for cakes or drinks.

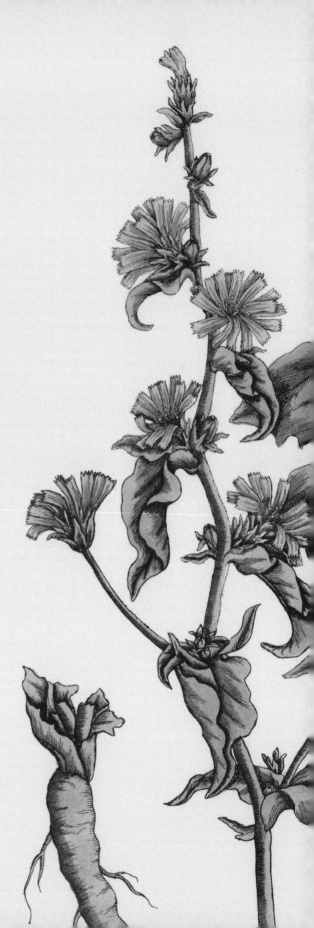

CORIANDER
Coriandrum sativum, Apiaceae family

Fresh-leaved, earthy-seeded, aromatic coriander is as present in the history of herbals as it is in many global cuisines today. Theophrastus discusses how to grow its seeds. Dioscorides records it as beneficial for skin infections, kidney stones and as a remedy for 'scrofulous' tumours (glandular swellings). Pliny provides various recipes using leaves and seeds, including a way to delay menstruation, while Avicenna pays homage to coriander's medicinal and culinary properties but warns against ingesting too much. It's an acquired taste but one that has certainly stood the test of time.

❧ **THE DESCRIPTION** John Gerard's 'very stinking herbe' (*Herball*, 1597) is similarly described by Mrs M. Grieve (*A Modern Herbal*, 1931) as 'intensely foetid', albeit a 'bright green, shining, glabrous [smooth]' herb with 'delicately pretty', 'pale mauve, almost white' flowers in 'shortly-stalked umbels'. Coriander's divided leaflets are similar to those of parsley or chervil and it produces clusters of round, woody seeds.

❧ **THE NAME** *Kopiavvov* (Theophrastus), *Koriannon* (Dioscorides) and *Kuzbara* (Avicenna) are all ancient, possibly scent-related names for coriander, and are the basis of its common and botanical name. The genus *Coriandrum* includes the widely cultivated *Coriandrum sativum* and the wilder *Coriandrum tordylium*, *sativum* being the Latin word for 'cultivated'. In North America, the leafy herb is known as *cilantro*.

❧ **THE PLACE** Thought to be native to the Eastern Mediterranean and Pakistan, coriander has been cultivated around the world for thousands of years and was imported into Britain by the Romans. It is now naturalised across much of Europe, Asia, Africa, South America, and parts of North America. It prefers fertile, well-drained soil, in full sun if growing for seeds, in partial shade if harvesting leaves. Limit watering.

❧ **THE TIME** Mrs M. Grieve advises starting off seeds in early spring under glass or outdoors in mid-spring if dry. 'The seeds are slow in germinating', she notes, and indeed Theophrastus advised soaking them before sowing. Pluck fresh leaves when the stems are around 15cm (6in) long. Harvest seeds in autumn by placing seedheads in a paper bag and hanging upside down for three weeks.

❧ **THE VIRTUES** Best known for its cooling and digestive properties, coriander was historically used to treat such terrible medieval skin-infections or diseases as St Anthony's fire and scrofula or the swollen-necked King's Evil. Coriander is now known to be rich in vitamins and minerals and as an essential oil is antibacterial and antifungal. The citrusy leaves and seeds are also delicious in a range of dishes.

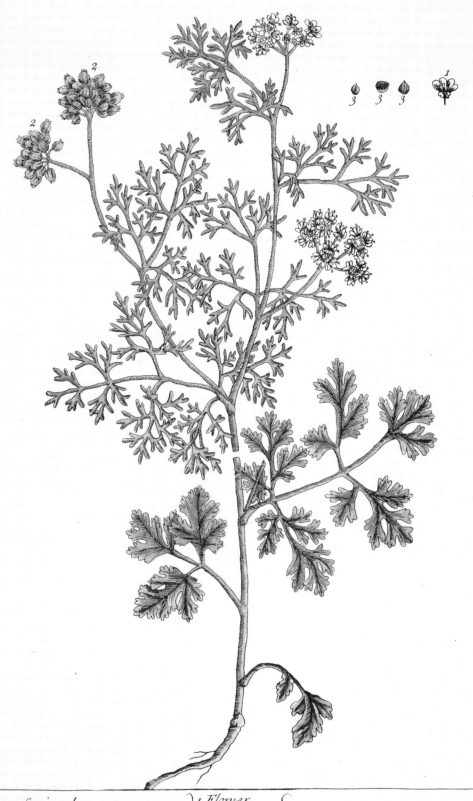

Plate 176.

1

2

2

3   3   3

Coriander.

Eliz. Blackwell delin. sculp. et Pinx.

1. Flower.
2. Seed Vessel.
3. Seed.

Coriandrum.

HEAL LEMON AND CORIANDER SOUP

This traditional Indo-Chinese soup combines vitamin-C-rich ingredients such as coriander, lemon, carrots and cabbage to create an immune-boosting, palate-cleansing and delicious broth, ideal for sipping during a fever or cold.

Serves 4
1 bunch of coriander
2.5cm (1in) cube fresh ginger
¼ head white or green cabbage
1 medium carrot
1 small green chilli
2 tbsp vegetable oil
1 tbsp cornflour or gram (chickpea) flour
1 litre (4 cups) vegetable stock
7–8 whole peppercorns
Juice of 1 lemon
Salt to taste

1 Wash the coriander, finely chop the stems and set the leaves aside. Peel and grate the ginger, shred the cabbage, finely slice the carrot and de-seed and slice the chilli.

2 Gently sauté the coriander stems and ginger in the oil until translucent. Add the cornflour or gram flour and stir for 2–3 minutes.

3 Pour in the stock and add the cabbage, carrot and chilli. Bring to a boil.

4 Stir in the peppercorns, lemon juice and salt to taste. Turn off the heat.

5 Tear the coriander leaves into the broth, ladle into bowls and serve immediately.

Other uses
❖ Add coriander essential oil to a citrusy massage oil blend to warm muscles.
❖ Drink a digestive infusion made with ½ tsp each of coriander, cumin and fennel seeds.

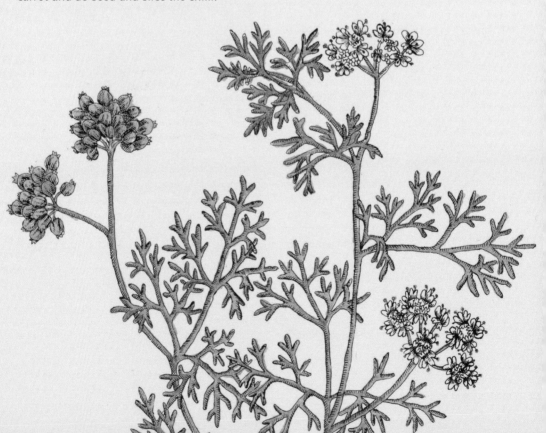

NOURISH *MOJO VERDE* (GREEN SAUCE)

Also known as *mojo de cilantro*, this Spanish, coriander-based green sauce hails from the Canary Island of Tenerife where it is traditionally served with *papas arrugadas* (miniature salt-crusted jacket potatoes). For a spicy kick, add a little fresh chilli to the mix.

Serves 4
1 garlic clove
1 tsp sea salt
¼ tsp ground cumin (optional)
1 large bunch of coriander
1 green chilli (optional)
125ml (½ cup) extra virgin olive oil
2 tbsp sherry vinegar or red wine vinegar

1 Chop the garlic and place in a pestle and mortar with the sea salt. Add the cumin, if desired, and grind.

2 Chop the coriander, add to the mix and pound further until combined. Incorporate a de-seeded and chopped green chilli if heat is desired.

3 Slowly pour in the oil, mashing until absorbed. Drizzle in the vinegar, gently stirring to mix.

4 Serve at room temperature.

Other uses
❖ Dry fry (without using oil) coriander seeds and use when pickling vegetables.
❖ Blend together ground coriander, cumin, chilli and turmeric for a curry powder base.

STYLE CORIANDER AND PINEAPPLE SORBET

The refreshing, cooling taste and smell of coriander leaves is perfect in a juice or sorbet. Coriander pairs particularly well with zingy fruits such as pineapple, lemon and lime. Add a stylish pop of brilliant green by serving the sorbet in frozen lime halves.

Serves 4
4 limes
1 fresh pineapple
Large handful of fresh coriander leaves
450g (2 cups) white caster sugar
1½ tsp lemon juice
Coriander sprigs, to serve

1 Halve and juice the limes. Remove and discard the lime flesh and place the empty shells in the freezer to set.

2 Peel, core and chop the pineapple into small pieces. Place in a blender with the coriander leaves and puree.

3 Place the sugar in a pan with 500ml (2 cups) of water and bring to a boil. Simmer until the sugar is dissolved. Remove from the heat.

4 Stir the pineapple purée, lime juice and lemon juice into the syrup. Leave to cool.

5 Strain and churn in an ice-cream maker according to instructions, then freeze in a suitable container. Or freeze in a lidded bowl for 3 hours until hard on the outside and slushy inside, then beat with a whisk and freeze for a further 4 hours.

6 Scoop the finished sorbet into the frozen lime shells for serving immediately. Garnish with coriander sprigs. Refreeze the remainder of the sorbet for later use.

Other uses
❖ Zing up a springtime brunch menu with an elegant tumbler of bright green coriander-lemon detox juice.
❖ A few drops of coriander essential oil on a melting candle imparts a welcoming scent.

SAFFRON
Crocus sativus, Iridaceae family

Saffron is the world's most valuable spice by weight owing to the labour-intensive growing and harvesting process. The thin, crimson threads, now mainly used to add earthy colour and flavour to paella, jewelled rice, *kahwa* tea and saffron buns, are actually the female stigmas of the purple-flowered, autumn-blooming saffron crocus (*Crocus sativus*). Although evidence shows that saffron has been cultivated for over three thousand years – most famously used by Cleopatra in a beautifying saffron-infused milk bath – its history goes back even further with traces of saffron recently found in cave art pigments dating back 50,000 years.

❧ THE DESCRIPTION True saffron (*Crocus sativus*) should not be confused with highly toxic *Colchicum autumnale*, also known as wild or meadow saffron. Both grow from corms but *Crocus sativus* has grass-like foliage that appears after flowering and its lilac-hued blooms have three distinctive, deep red stigmas. The more robust *Colchicum autumnale* has larger, floppier, spring leaves followed by goblet-shaped pinker flowers.

❧ THE NAME The genus name *Crocus* has its roots in the Greek word *Krokos*, the Hebrew/Roman *karkom* and the Arabic *kurkum*, coined specifically to describe saffron. The species name *sativus* pays homage to saffron's extensive history as a 'cultivated' plant, while the ancient Arabic *Zahafaran* (John Gerard, *Herball*, 1597) or *Zarparan* meaning 'flower with golden petals' inspired the common name of this prized spice.

❧ THE PLACE It is hard to pinpoint saffron's exact origins although the most likely region appears to be Greece and the plant's ancestor is probably the wild crocus species *Crocus cartwrightianus*. Saffron is still cultivated in Greece and the saffron crocus has since naturalised in the Czech Republic, Slovakia, Iran, Italy, Morocco, Pakistan, Spain, Turkey and the West Himalayas. To grow, plant corms in a sunny, free-draining site in a border or container.

❧ THE TIME The *Crocus* genus has species that flower in autumn, winter and spring and saffron is the most familiar autumn-flowering form. Saffron does not produce viable seeds so to propagate, divide clumps in spring before corms get overcrowded. Saffron stigmas should be harvested mid-morning on a sunny day when flowers are in full bloom, then allow to dry on a paper towel before storing in an airtight container.

❧ THE VIRTUES Saffron was traditionally 'esteemed a great Cordial, Strenthening ye Heart & vital Spirits, resisting Putrefactions & usefull in all Kinds of malignant & contagious Distempers, Fevers, Small Pox & Measles' (Elizabeth Blackwell, *A Curious Herbal*, 1737–39). A powerful antioxidant rich in carotenoids, it has been used since antiquity to beautify, enhance memory, improve eyesight, spice foods and as a yellow dye.

Plate 144.

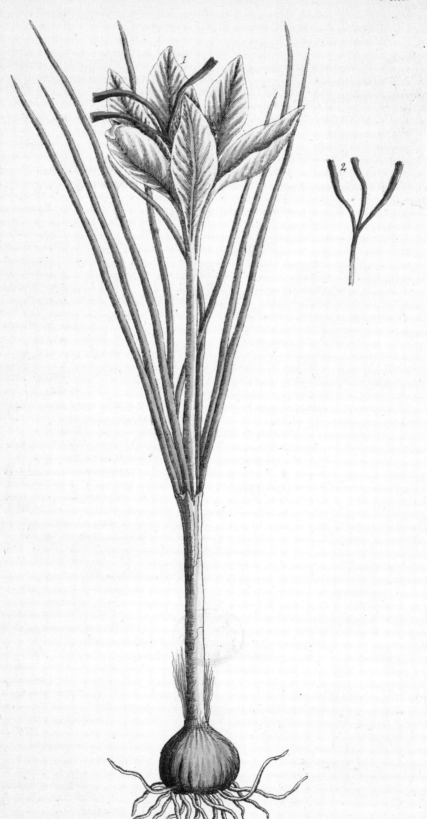

Saffron

Eliz. Blackwell delin. sculp. et Pinx.

{ 1. Flower.
{ 2. Stamina.

Crocus.

HEAL
KAHWA TEA

Warming saffron tea is traditionally served in parts of India at celebration dinners or after food, but can also be imbibed to lift the spirits, build immunity, improve digestion or help beat a cold. Made with or without green tea, carotenoid-rich saffron also adds a gorgeous amber colour and an earthy scent plus brain-boosting vitamin B.

Serves 4
4–5 saffron threads
3 green bruised cardamom pods
1 cinnamon stick
2 tbsp blanched flaked almonds
4 tsp honey

1 Combine the saffron, cardamom pods and cinnamon stick in a pan with 750ml (3 cups) of water. Bring to a boil. Simmer gently for 2–3 minutes until the water is golden amber.

2 Divide the almonds and honey between four tea glasses or small cups.

3 Pour tea on top, stir gently and drink while warm.

Other uses
❧ Infuse 100ml (3½fl oz) of sweet almond oil with 10–15 strands of saffron for a week to create a complexion-enhancing facial oil.
❧ Add a few strands of antioxidant-rich saffron and 3 drops of lavender essential oil to a bowl of hot water for a pore-opening facial steam.

NOURISH
PERSIAN JEWELLED RICE

Just a few strands of saffron are needed to turn plain white rice into ochre-tinted, earthy *paella* or Persian jewelled rice.

Serves 6
4–5 saffron threads
80ml (1/3 cup) boiled water
50g (1¾oz) pistachios
Small handful of fresh flat leaf parsley
300g (1½ cups) basmati rice
3 tbsp unsalted butter
8 green cardamom pods
2 cinnamon sticks
2 bay leaves
80g (3oz) dried cranberries or barberries
50g (1¾oz) dried apricots, chopped
2 tbsp pomegranate seeds
Zest of 1 orange
Salt and black pepper to taste

1 Infuse the saffron in the boiled water for about 1 hour.

2 Lightly toast the pistachios, wash and chop the parsley and rinse the rice of all starch.

3 Melt 1 tbsp of the butter in a large lidded pan. Stir in the cardamom, cinnamon sticks, rice, bay leaves and a little salt.

4 Pour in 750ml (3 cups) of water. Cover and cook on low heat for 12 minutes, then set aside for 5 minutes. Fluff and divide into two portions.

5 Add the saffron water and 1 tbsp of butter to one half of the rice. Add the pistachios, dried fruit, pomegranate seeds, orange zest and parsley, remaining butter and salt and pepper to the other half. Mix the two rices together and serve.

Other uses
❧ Blend yogurt, minced garlic, lemon juice, olive oil and and a saffron infusion (see page 18) to create a tangy dip.
❧ Saffron adds a warming, golden element to cakes, custard or rice pudding.

STYLE
SAFFRON NEGRONI

Add a dash of sensual saffron syrup to spice up a dry Negroni and intensify its sunset colour.

Makes 1 Negroni
To make the saffron syrup:
5 saffron threads
5 green cardamom pods
200g (1 cup) granulated sugar
Zest and juice of 2 limes

To make the saffron Negroni:
40ml (1½fl oz) Campari
40ml (1½fl oz) gin
40ml (1½fl oz) vermouth
2 tbsp saffron syrup (see above)
2–3 cracked ice cubes
Zest of 1 orange (peeled into thin curls)
2 extra saffron threads to garnish

1 Combine the saffron, cardamom and sugar and lime juice and zest in a pan with 185ml (¾ cup) of water. Bring to a boil. Simmer until syrupy. Leave to cool.

2 Place the Campari, gin and vermouth in a cocktail shaker. Add 2 tbsp of cooled syrup and shake gently.

3 Place the ice in a 200ml (7fl oz) martini or old-fashioned glass and pour the saffron Negroni mix over the top.

4 Garnish with the orange zest and saffron.

Other uses
❧ Plant saffron (*Crocus sativus*) around the garden for gorgeous autumn colour.
❧ The Romans placed saffron on the marital bed to enhance love. Extend the tradition by gifting sachets of saffron to a bride and groom, or as a wedding favour for guests.

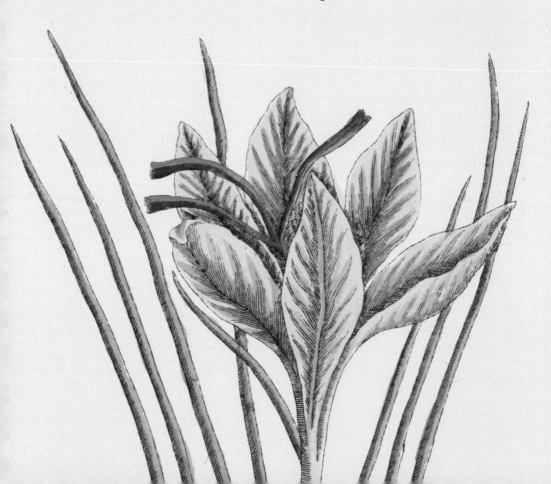

FENNEL
Foeniculum vulgare, Apiaceae family

Common, garden or wild fennel (*Foeniculum vulgare*) is one of the most handsome herbs around, producing a tower of feathery leaves and flat umbels of golden flowers followed by sweet, anise-flavoured oblong fruits known as fennel seeds. Prized by the ancient Greeks as a culinary and medicinal herb – particularly as an appetite suppressant – it was introduced and widely cultivated by the Romans who used it for treating ailments from stomach issues to the stings of scorpions and serpents. This staple and stately perennial has remained popular right through to the present day.

❀ **THE DESCRIPTION** Herbal accounts dating back to Dioscorides, Theophrastus and Pliny appear to describe several types of fennel, most of which are variations of *Foeniculum vulgare*. Key varieties include the gorgeous bronze-leaved fennel (*Foeniculum vulgare* 'Purpureum') and Florence fennel or Finocchio (*Foeniculum vulgare* var. *dulce*), also cultivated for its edible, bulbous stem-base.

❀ **THE NAME** Fennel's present-day species name *vulgare* was validated by the English botanist Philip Miller in *The Gardener's Dictionary* (1768). The genus name *Foeniculum* – first used by the Romans and corrupted into the common name fennel – derives from the Latin word *foenum* or *fenum* meaning 'hay', which could refer to its aroma, seeds or leaf structure.

❀ **THE PLACE** The herbaceous perennial is native to much of the Mediterranean, Eurasia and northern Africa, but has been introduced to large swathes of more northerly Europe, Asia, southern Africa, west coast North America and Central and South America. Common fennel prefers a sunny spot in light, free-draining soil. Florence fennel is grown as an annual vegetable and prefers fertile, well-drained soil. Earth up around bulbs as they swell.

❀ **THE TIME** Sow common fennel in mid-spring in situ when all threat of frost has passed. Sow Florence fennel under cover in mid-spring or direct in summer. In both cases, harvest the feathery fronds from spring to autumn. Fennel seeds can be eaten fresh as soon as they are ripe or dried for year-round use. Harvest Florence fennel bulbs around 20 days after earthing up.

❀ **THE VIRTUES** As noted by Elizabeth Blackwell (*A Curious Herbal*, 1737–39), fennel 'leaves are said to encrease Nurse's Milk & strengthen the Sight, and are good for the Stone and Gravel' while 'The seed is carminative, expelling Wind, strengthening the Bowels and helping the Collic'. Fennel tea is still a popular drink, the seeds and fragrant essential oil are taken to support digestion, and all parts taste delicious.

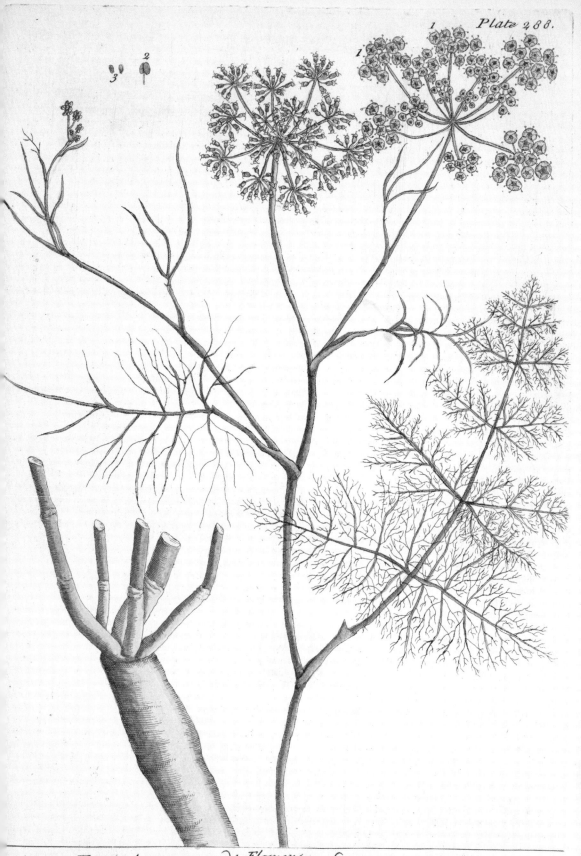

Fennel.

Eliz. Blackwell delin. sculp. et Pinx.

1. *Flowers.*
2. *Seed Joind.*
3. *Seed separate.*

Foeniculum.

Plate 288.

HEAL *MUKHWAS* (FENNEL BREATH FRESHENER)

Fennel seeds – the core ingredient of the Indian post-meal snack *mukhwas* – are naturally sweet, a digestive aid and palate-cleansing. Add high-fibre, high-protein sesame and flax seeds to further stimulate digestion and help keep hunger pangs at bay.

Makes 1 x 250ml (9fl oz) jar
4 tbsp fennel seeds
4 tbsp white sesame seeds
4 tbsp black sesame seeds
4 tbsp flax seeds
1–2 tbsp lemon juice
Salt to taste

1 Mix all the seeds in a bowl.

2 Add the lemon juice and a pinch of salt. Stir well, cover the bowl with a cloth and set aside for 1 hour.

3 Dry roast the mixture in a preheated non-stick pan, stirring continuously until an aroma is released.

4 Remove the pan from the heat and allow the mixture to cool.

5 Store finished *mukhwas* in an airtight sterilised 250ml (9fl oz) glass lidded jar.

Other uses
❖ Fennel tea is particularly good for digestion, relieving water retention and wind, or to help increase milk flow for nursing mothers.
❖ Massage 2–3 drops of fennel essential oil diluted in 1 tbsp of sweet almond oil onto the stomach to help soothe and detoxify. Avoid during pregancy.

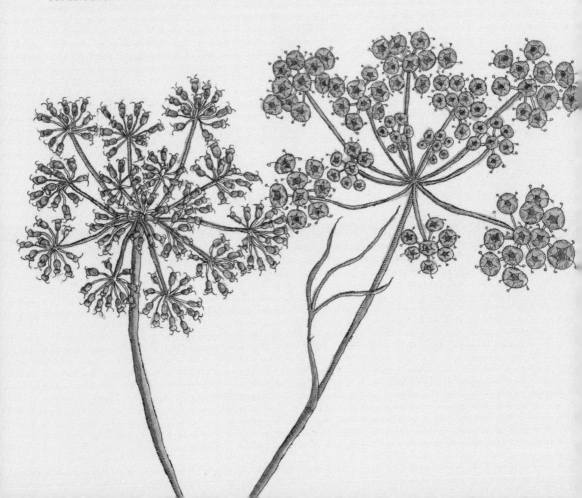

NOURISH *MARATHOKEF-TEDES* (FENNEL FRITTERS)

This traditional Greek snack is a lovely use of sweet, anise-flavoured fennel bulbs and fronds, traditionally served up with drinks and a side helping of yogurt. The dish is named after the Ancient Greek word *marathos* meaning fennel, the ancient battle site of Marathon being 'a place full of fennels'.

Makes about 12 fritters
4 small fennel bulbs with fronds attached
8 spring onions
Large handful of fresh parsley
Small handful of fresh dill
150g (1 heaped cup) plain flour
250ml (1 cup) olive oil
Sea salt and pepper to taste
Lemon wedges, to serve

1 Wash and chop the fennel fronds, spring onions, parsley and dill. Finely slice the fennel bulbs. Combine in a large bowl.

2 Season with salt and pepper and sift in the flour. Add 125ml (½ cup) of water and stir until the mixture can be shaped into 12 evenly sized balls. Flatten into patties using your hands.

3 Pour enough oil into a large pan to cover the base and then heat until sizzling. Cook two or three fritters at a time, 4 minutes each side, pressing down with a spatula until evenly crispy and golden.

4 Rest the fritters on a paper towel to remove excess oil. Serve with lemon wedges.

Other uses
❧ Slow roast fennel bulbs in a little olive oil to bring out the natural sweetness and serve with slices of orange and goat's cheese.
❧ Swirl an intense pop of fennel pollen – harvested fresh from upside-down flower heads tapped into a paper bag, or store-bought – into cream, add to a dry-roasting spice rub, or sprinkle onto fresh fruit or cakes.

STYLE FENNEL AND GRAPEFRUIT BODY WASH

Imbue a homemade body wash with the uplifting yet comforting scent and detoxifying, nourishing properties of fennel essential oil. Pair with zesty citrus essential oils such as lemon, sweet orange or grapefruit plus skin-smoothing coconut, jojoba or sweet almond oil for a pampering, refreshing start to the day. For a lovely gift, add a natural card label embellished with a pressed fennel flower.

Makes 1 x 500ml (17½fl oz) bottle
375ml (1½ cups) unscented liquid castile soap (preferably organic)
8 tbsp raw runny honey
2 tbsp fractionated (liquid) coconut oil, jojoba oil or sweet almond oil
2 tsp vitamin E or wheatgerm oil
40 drops grapefruit essential oil
30 drops fennel essential oil

1 Place all the ingredients in a jug. Mix well with a spoon or wooden stick. If a little more scent is desired add a few more drops of essential oil.

2 Decant into a 500ml (17½fl oz) amber glass or fully recyclable PET plastic pump top bottle.

Other uses
❧ Press fennel flowers into discs of air-drying clay to leave a pretty impression – seal and glaze to use as ornaments.
❧ Leave fennel seedheads in place to add ornamental interest to a winter garden and provide a nutritious treat for birds.

LIQUORICE
Glycyrrhiza glabra, Fabaceae family

Used as a sweetener as well as a digestive by the ancient Greeks, Egyptians, Persians and Romans, today liquorice (*Glycyrrhiza*) is so closely associated with confectionery that it's easy to forget that its edible roots have been used for centuries as a medicine. Now mainly grown in the Mediterranean and Asia, this bushy, purple-flowered, deep-rooted legume was once cultivated in Britain, most famously in Pontefract, Yorkshire, after being introduced by 11th-century Crusaders from the Middle East. It was certainly known to Geoffrey Chaucer, who wove the herb into his raunchy *The Miller's Tale* (1380–90).

❧ THE DESCRIPTION Liquorice hails from the roots of *Glycyrrhiza glabra* (European liquorice), *G. echinata* (hedgehog liquorice), *G. uralensis* or *G. inflata* (Chinese liquorice) and *G. lepidota* (American licorice). European liquorice has 'light, spreading, pinnate foliage, presenting an almost feathery appearance from a distance' (Mrs M. Grieve, *A Modern Herbal*, 1931), with pale, purple-tinged, pea-like flowers.

❧ THE NAME The genus *Glycyrrhiza* stems from the Greek word *Glyrrhiza* used by Dioscorides in *De Materia Medica* (AD 50–70) to describe a sweet (*glukos*) root (*riza*). The specific name *glabra* refers to the 'smooth' fruit pods of this species in comparison to its spikier relatives. The word liquorice – or licorice as it is also spelled – derives from the Latin botanical name *Liquiritia*, a corruption of *Glyrrhiza*.

❧ THE PLACE Herbalists such as Nicholas Culpeper, John Parkinson and Elizabeth Blackwell record liquorice as a field and garden plant with John Gerard boasting that his garden 'has plenty'. While not widely cultivated as an ornamental today, it can be grown in deep, fertile, well-drained soil, faring best in its native southern Europe, as well as the Middle East and parts of Asia.

❧ THE TIME This herbaceous perennial flowers in midsummer, fruits in autumn and dies back in winter. To harvest the roots, it's necessary to wait until the third or fourth year of growth when the plant has become bushy and the roots are a good size. To grow from seed, start off under glass indoors in spring or autumn, or divide mature plants in the autumn.

❧ THE VIRTUES Liquorice roots are now known to contain *glycyrrhizin*, which is substantially sweeter than sugar. It can be extracted via a decoction (see page 18) of the roots and used as a culinary flavouring or natural sweetener. The roots can also be chewed to help clean teeth, or used whole or powdered to make a digestive tea. Use moderately: liquorice can raise blood pressure, affect heart rhythms and have a laxative effect, so avoid if you have a history of heart disease and high blood pressure.

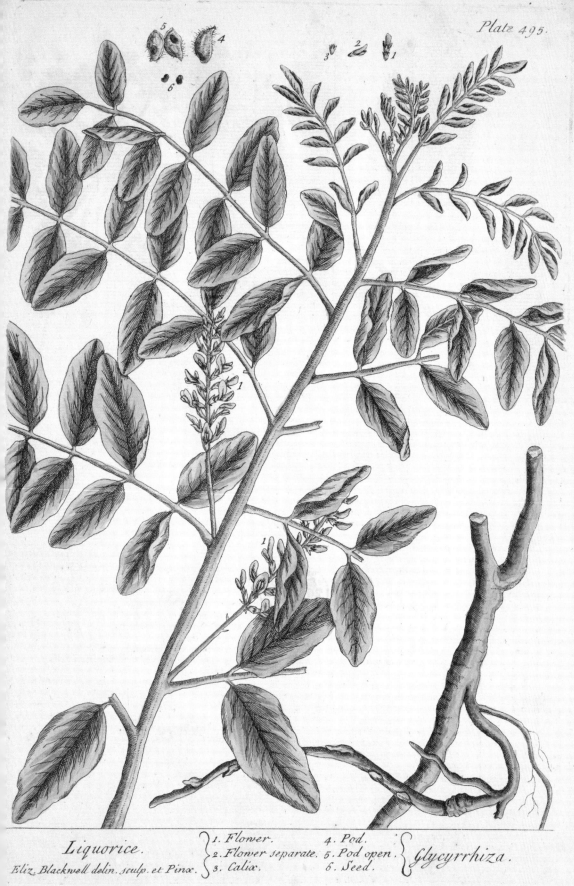

Platz 495.

Liquorice.

Eliz. Blackwell delin. sculp. et Pinx.

1. Flower.
2. Flower separate.
3. Calix.
4. Pod.
5. Pod open.
6. Seed.

Glycyrrhiza.

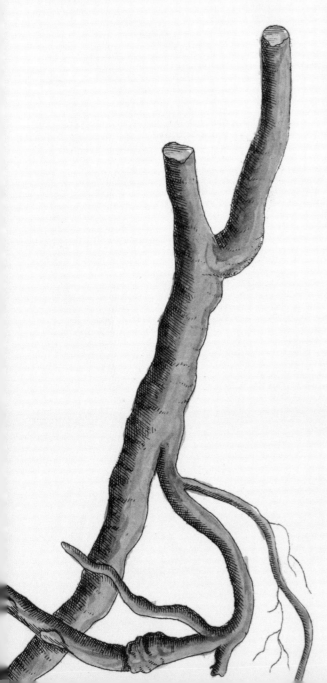

HEAL
LIQUORICE TOOTHBRUSH

Naturally antibacterial, soft, fibrous
liquorice root has been chewed for
millennia to keep teeth clean. Use
moderately, morning and night as part
of a regular dental routine, after meals
to help freshen breath or as a helpful aid
when quitting smoking.

Makes 1 brush
**1 fresh liquorice root around 18cm (7in) long
by 1cm (½in) diameter**

1 Select a store-bought or homegrown
liquorice root that is fairly straight and not
too thick.

2 Chew on one end until the outer root bark
becomes loose. Discard the bark.

3 Continue to chew lightly until the inner
root fibres start to resemble a brush. Gently
rub over each tooth and gumline to clean
away dirt and plaque.

4 Replace liquorice stick when dry,
tasteless, or too short to handle.

Other uses
❀ Occasionally sip on a decoction of
liquorice root tea to help with digestive
issues, inflammation or stress.
❀ Make your own sore-throat lozenges from
liquorice root tea, slippery elm bark powder
and honey.

NOURISH
LIQUORICE ENERGY BALLS

The *umami* flavour of liquorice can be used to add colour and body to a range of sweet and savoury dishes. Try rolling date (or fig) and nut balls in liquorice powder for a naturally sweet, energy-boosting snack. Eat in moderation.

Makes 30 balls
200g (7oz) stoned dates or dried figs
100g (3½oz) nuts such as blanched almonds
   or cashews
2 tbsp ground liquorice root

1 Place the dates or figs, nuts and 1 tbsp of water in a food processor and blend until mixed.

2 Transfer to a bowl and form into small, bite-sized balls with your hands.

3 Place the liquorice in a saucer and roll the balls in the powder until lightly coated.

4 Store in an airtight container in the fridge.

Other uses
❧ Add a liquorice powder and sea-salt twist to a classic crème brulée served with caramelised figs or poached pears.
❧ Place a liquorice root stick or two in a pot roast, or combine ground liquorice root into a roasting rub.

STYLE
LIQUORICE CANDY

Decorative paper bags or glass jars of traditional liquorice-flavoured candy shapes or sticks make perfect sweet treats or gifts. Eat in moderation.

Makes approx. 100 small candy portions
340g (1 cup) molasses or honey
250g (1¼ cups) raw sugar
115g (½ cup) butter
2 tsp ground liquorice root
1 tsp ground anise
90g (¾ cup) plain flour
½ tsp Himalayan pink salt
1 tsp black food colouring

1 Place the molasses or honey, sugar, butter, ground liquorice and ground anise in a double boiler. Bring to a boil until the temperature reaches 115°C (240°F). A tsp of the mixture dropped into cold water should form a ball.

2 Remove from the heat, quickly sift in the flour and add the salt and food colouring. Stir, allow to cool slightly and knead into a soft dough. Roll into a sausage, wrap in baking parchment and place in a fridge to cool for several hours until set.

3 Remove from the baking parchment and cut, or tear and mould into liquorice candy shapes. Wrap each candy piece in baking parchment and place in a paper bag or jar.

4 Store in the fridge for up to 2 weeks.

Other uses
❧ Bushy liquorice plants at the back of deep borders provide a lovely backdrop for shorter plants.
❧ Use earthy liquorice root as a rustic garnish for anise-flavoured cocktails made with spirits such as Pernod, pastis, anisette, absinthe, ouzo or sambuca.

HYSSOP
Hyssopus officinalis, Lamiaceae family

Today, hyssop's medicinal qualities may be outweighed by the ornamental and aromatic appeal of its blue, pink or white-spired flowers and dark green, lance-shaped leaves. Yet this ancient herb has expectorant, antiseptic and soothing properties that are useful for easing coughs and sore throats as well as a lovely floral-mint flavour. Although 'hyssop' is mentioned in the Bible as a cleansing herb, scholars are divided on whether this is *Hyssopus officinalis* or other plant species fitting the given description, such as Syrian oregano (*Origanum syriacum*) or the caper plant (*Capparis spinosa*).

❧ THE DESCRIPTION The forms of this 'evergreen bushy herb, growing to 1–2 feet high, with square stem, linear leaves and flowers in whorls, six- to fifteen-flowered' (Mrs M. Grieve, *A Modern Herbal*, 1931) bloom in different shades: *Hyssopus officinalis* is blue, *H. officinalis* f. *albus* white, and *H. officinalis* 'Roseus' pink. Each tiny flower, on close inspection, is two-lipped and tubular and the leaves are semi-evergreen.

❧ THE NAME Not to be confused with similarly aromatic and flavoursome anise hyssop (*Agastache foeniculum*) – which is confusingly neither hyssop nor anise (*Pimpinella anisum*) – true hyssop (*Hyssopus officinalis*) traces its genus name back to the Greek word *Hyssopus* and the Hebrew *esov* or *esob*, used to describe a sacred plant. *Officinalis* references hyssop's use as a medicinal herb.

❧ THE PLACE Native to the Mediterranean and Western Asia, as well as parts of Europe, Caucasus and the Middle East, hyssop has also become naturalised elsewhere, including the United States where it was cultivated by American colonists. Grow in chalky or loamy, well-drained soil in full sun, pairing with catmint, lavender and rosemary as suggested by Mrs M. Grieve (*A Modern Herbal*, 1931).

❧ THE TIME Harvest hyssop leaves year-round (in sheltered, warmer climes) and pick blooms from mid-to-late summer for drying, making a fresh infusion, or adding a pinch to soups, stews or salads. Propagate by seed or softwood cuttings in summer and leave seedheads in place through autumn, winter and early spring as food for the birds.

❧ THE VIRTUES Throat infections, phlegm, lung disease, a weak stomach, jaundice, bruises, wounds, toothache, worms and lice are just some of the ailments herbalists listed as treatable by hyssop, in the form of a decoction, oxymel or poultice. Figs and wine were also offered to help the medicine go down. Hyssop essential oil is now known to be antiseptic and the chopped leaves add a bittersweet flavour to dishes.

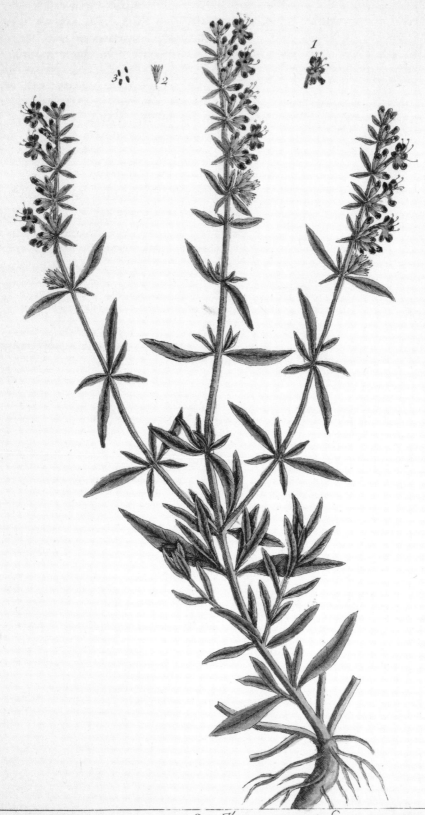

Plate 296.

Hyssop.

1. Flower separate.
2. Calix.
3. Seed.

Hyssopus.

Eliz. Blackwell delin. sculp. et Pinx.

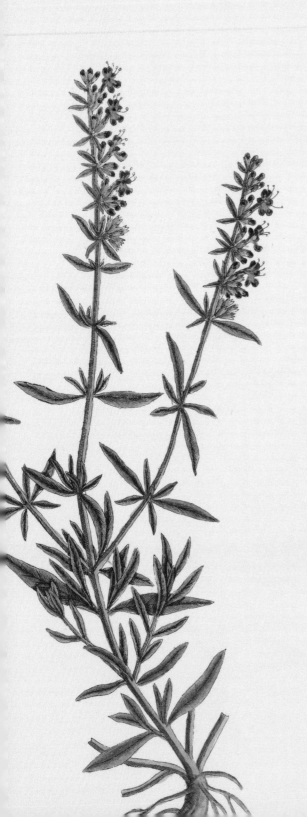

HEAL
HYSSOP OXYMEL

Create a traditional wintertime oxymel – a combination of herb-infused honey and vinegar – with hyssop and activating apple cider vinegar to help reduce fever and ease congestion. Avoid while pregnant.

Makes 1 x 500ml (17½fl oz) jar
12g (½ cup) dried hyssop leaves
250ml (¾ cup) organic honey
250ml (1 cup) apple cider vinegar

1 Quarter fill a 500ml (17½fl oz) sterilised glass jar with the leaves.

2 Pour in the honey and vinegar until almost full – leave room for shaking.

3 Stir the mixture with a clean, dry spoon. Seal with a non-corrosive lid.

4 Shake well until all the ingredients are mixed. Store in a cool dry place.

5 Shake every 2–3 days for 2 weeks, then strain and pour into another 500ml (17½fl oz) sterilised glass jar.

6 Take 1 tbsp of hyssop oxymel a day to keep a cold at bay, to ease a cough as required, or dissolve in 250ml (1 cup) of just-boiled water to use as a soothing infusion.

Other uses
❖ Make a decongestant chest rub for a chesty cold using 10 drops of hyssop essential oil in 1–2 tbsp of sweet almond oil.
❖ Treat a bruise or small cut with a poultice of mashed fresh hyssop leaves held in place with a bandage.

NOURISH
HYSSOP-GLAZED CARROTS

Bitter, slightly minty hyssop leaves pair beautifully with sweet carrots in this simple yet delicious glazed side dish – a great way to welcome early spring carrots to the menu.

Serves 4
450g (1lb) baby carrots
250ml (1 cup) vegetable stock
1 tbsp honey
1 tsbp unsalted butter
2 tbsp finely chopped fresh hyssop leaves
Salt and freshly ground white pepper to taste

1 Peel the carrots and slice into thin batons, or if very young leave whole.

2 Combine the carrots, stock, honey, butter and a pinch of salt and pepper in a pan. Simmer over a medium heat for around 20 minutes until the carrots are tender and the liquid syrupy.

3 Turn off the heat. Sprinkle 1 tbsp of the chopped hyssop over the glazed carrots. Gently toss.

4 Transfer to a serving dish, sprinkle over the remaining hyssop and eat while warm.

Other uses
❧ Infuse Mediterranean-style soups or sauces with a little dried hyssop tied in a muslin sachet, as the dry, brittle leaves can be sharp.
❧ Hyssop also pairs well with sweet stone fruits such as peaches, or can be infused into custard or ice cream – use flowers, which are less pungent than leaves.

STYLE
HYSSOP RITUAL BATH

It may or may not be the holy hyssop mentioned in the Bible but the herb's cleansing and restorative powers are perfect for an energy-aligning, fragrant ritual bath.

Makes 1 bath bag
1 muslin drawstring sachet bag
6 tbsp dried hyssop leaves and flowers
500g (2½ cups) Epsom salts
3 tbsp sweet almond oil
2 drops hyssop essential oil
2 drops lemongrass essential oil
2 drops lavender essential oil
Candles and healing crystals (optional)

1 Fill a muslin sachet bag with the hyssop leaves and flowers. pull drawstring to close.

2 Place the Epsom salts in a 500ml (17½fl oz) lidded glass jar, followed by the almond oil and essential oils. Seal and shake gently to combine.

3 Run a warm bath. Place the hyssop bath sachet under the running tap.

4 Add a cupful of the aromatic bath salts, stirring with hands until dissolved.

5 Place healing crystals such as quartz or amethyst in the bath and light the candles.

6 Soak for at least 20 minutes, breathing deeply to inhale the infused steam, and use the bag to wash and soothe skin.

Other uses
❧ Hang bunches of dried hyssop leaves and flowers around the house as a natural air freshener.
❧ Plant hyssop in the garden to attract bees and other pollinators and use the flower spires in bouquets.

JASMINE
Jasminum officinale, Oleaceae family

Jasmine is best known for its heady, evocative scent – much loved and utilised to beautify, heal and impart flavour for thousands of years. This sweet fragrance is emitted by the white, star-shaped flowers of many of the plants in the 200-strong *Jasminum* genus and of these, the most cultivated species are common jasmine (*Jasminum officinale*), Spanish jasmine (*J. grandiflorum*) and Arabian jasmine (*J. sambac*). Grown for its essential oil, used in perfumery and to restore balance and ease stress, jasmine also makes a beautiful ornamental climber.

❧ THE DESCRIPTION As noted by Nicholas Culpeper (*Complete Herbal*, 1653), 'Jessamine' is 'a tree or shrub, shooting out long, slender, green twigs or branches … with long pinnated leaves, made of several, sharp-pointed pinnae, set opposite to each other with an odd one at the end', the flowers 'being longish tubes, spreading out at the top into five broad segments … of a white colour, and a pleasant agreeable smell'.

❧ THE NAME Most of jasmine's historical names, such as *Jessamine*, *Gessemine* and its Latinised genus name *Jasminum* stem from the Persian *Yasemin* or *Yasmin*. Common jasmine's species name *officinale* points to medicinal use, Spanish jasmine's *grandiflorum* to large flowers and Arabian jasmine's *sambac* to the Arabic word for jasmine, *Zambach*.

❧ THE PLACE The *Jasminum* or Jessamine described by Culpeper, John Gerard and Elizabeth Blackwell is native to a large sweep of Asia and the southern Caucasus but is now naturalised in parts of western Europe, the Mediterranean and North Africa. *J. sambac*, *J. auriculatum* and *J. grandiflorum* are more specific to parts of Asia, Africa and the Arabian Peninsula. All varieties of jasmine need fertile, well-drained soil and a sheltered spot in sun or light shade.

❧ THE TIME Common jasmine, unlike the yellow-flowered winter jasmine (*Jasminum nudiflorum*), blooms from midsummer to autumn and may need protection in regions with very cold winters. Jasmine flowers should be harvested in the late afternoon or early evening when scent is at its strongest. Propagate by taking semi-ripe cuttings in spring and summer or take hardwood cuttings in winter. Prune after flowering.

❧ THE VIRTUES 'The oil made by infusion of the flowers, is used much in perfumes' records Culpeper, although he also suggests that jasmine's strong scent may give those of a hot constitution a headache. Its fragrant oils are extracted via *enfleurage* (using odourless fat) or using solvents. Jasmine has also been used medicinally for a cough, to ease stress, and as a delicate flavouring for tea, rice and sweets.

Plate 13.

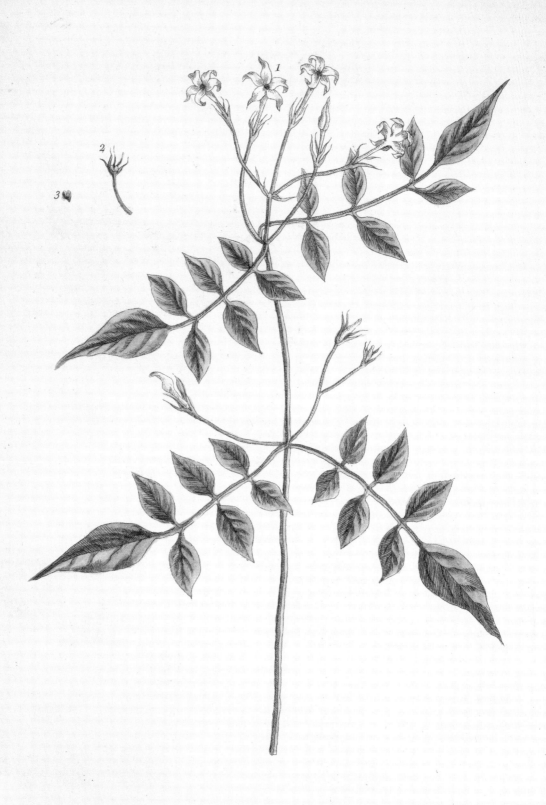

Jasmine
Eliz. Blackwell delin. sculp. et Pinx.

1 Flower
2 Fruit
3 Seed

Jasminum

HEAL
JASMINE BODY BUTTER

Harness the balancing, skin-rejuvenating, stress-busting properties of jasmine essential oil whipped up with nourishing shea butter, coconut oil and sweet almond oil to create an ideal body balm for stretch marks or skin requiring tone. Avoid during pregnancy.

Makes 1 x 250ml (8fl oz) wide-mouthed jar
100g (3½oz) shea butter
4 tbsp fractionated (liquid) coconut oil
2 tbsp sweet almond oil
Up to 5 drops jasmine absolute essential oil

1 Place the shea butter and coconut oil in a bowl over a pan of boiling water. Gently heat, stirring to combine. Remove from the heat and allow to cool.

2 Stir in the almond oil and jasmine oil and place in the fridge until almost solidified (approx. 1 hour).

3 Transfer to a mixing bowl and whip with a hand mixer until white and fluffy.

4 Decant into a 250ml (8fl oz) wide-mouthed, amber glass, screw-lid jar and seal. Use the body butter to smooth and soothe skin as desired.

Other uses
❧ Massage 2 drops of jasmine absolute essential oil diluted in 1 tbsp of sweet almond oil into pulse points to help beat insomnia, depression or stress. Avoid during pregnancy.
❧ Create a nourishing, shine-enhancing hair mask of crushed jasmine flowers, natural yogurt and coconut oil.

NOURISH
JASMINE TEA

Add an extra layer of ritual to jasmine tea by infusing your own batch with freshly picked jasmine blooms.

Makes 1 x 500ml (17½fl oz) jar or tea caddy
200g (2 cups) loose-leaf green tea
Several large handfuls of fresh jasmine flowers (just opened)

1 Spread the tea out on a large flat tray. Set to one side.

2 Harvest two large handfuls of jasmine flowers in the late afternoon, enough to create a layer over the tea. Leave in a warm place.

3 In the evening, when the fragrance is at its strongest, harvest more flowers. Remove the first batch of flowers, and discard, and spread the new batch over the tea. Leave overnight in a dry spot.

4 Remove the flowers the next evening and repeat steps 2 and 3 for a few days until the tea is fully infused, harvesting fresh blooms each time.

5 When the tea is adequately scented, remove the last batch of flowers and decant into a clean, airtight 500ml (17½fl oz) lidded jar or caddy.

6 To prepare jasmine tea, steep 1 tbsp of the infused tea in 250ml (1 cup) of just-boiled water for at least 5 minutes. Strain and serve while warm.

Other uses
❧ Cook Thai 'jasmine' rice in jasmine-infused tea to impart extra notes of the bloom after which this rice is named.
❧ An infusion of jasmine tea also adds a floral, exotic layer to chocolate ganache, chocolate truffles, chocolate mousse or rice pudding.

STYLE
SENSUAL CANDLE

Jasmine is a particularly relaxing, sensual choice for aromatherapy candles, by itself or with woody, citrus or floral scents such as cedarwood, sandalwood, vetiver, bergamot, patchouli or ylang ylang.

Makes 1 x 250ml (8fl oz) jar candle
150g (5oz) soy wax pellets
50g (1¾oz) beeswax pellets
1 metal-bottomed wick (plus optional wick holder)
1 (250ml/8fl oz) glass jar (vessel for candle)
4 drops jasmine absolute essential oil, plus extra for burning
20 drops cedarwood essential oil
10 drops bergamot essential oil

1 The weight of wax needed is 80 per cent of the volume of your vessel, which is 200g (7oz) of wax for a 250ml (8oz) jar.

2 Place the metal tab of a wick on the base of the jar and secure the cotton part with a wick holder or clothes peg balanced on the rim.

3 Place the pellets in a bowl over a pan of boiling water and melt until liquid. Remove from the heat and allow to cool to 140°C (285°F). Use a thermometer to check.

4 Gently mix in the essential oils (at a ratio of around 40–50 drops of essential oil per 225g (8oz) wax, although some oils such as jasmine absolute are stronger).

5 Carefully pour the wax into the jar and leave to cure for 2 days.

6 Light the candle, adding an extra drop of jasmine absolute essential oil to the top pool of melting wax for added scent.

Other uses
❧ Create a delicate *enfleurage* perfume by sandwiching successions of highly fragrant fresh jasmine flowers between coconut-oil smeared glass sheets – rub the flower-oil pomade directly onto pulse points or extract into a homemade eau de toilette using alcohol.
❧ Trail a fragrant climber of jasmine under a bedroom window for sweeter dreams, and a nutritious treat for birds.

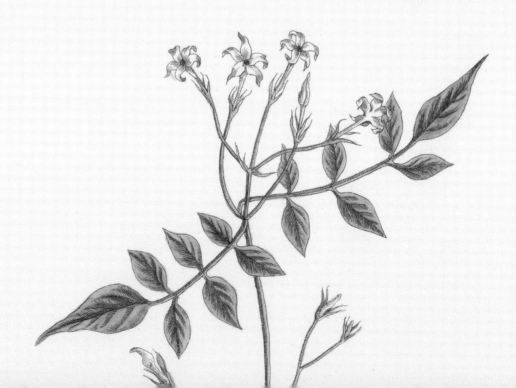

LAVENDER
Lavendula, Lamiaceae family

The calming, cleaning and perfuming qualities of lavender have been harnessed for thousands of years. Of the 50 or so species of this woody, aromatic perennial the most widely cultivated include English lavender (*Lavandula angustifolia* – shown opposite), spike lavender (*L. latifolia*) and French lavender (*L. stoechas*). Entering the gardens of England via medieval monasteries, lavender was soon placed among linens, prescribed for headaches, carried to ward off the Plague, and later became a hugely popular perfume. It remains one of the best-loved and most popular herbs.

❧ THE DESCRIPTION Narrow-leaved 'Lavandula' (*Lavandula angustifolia*) grows 'about two Foot high, the Leaves are a light Green and the Flowers bluish'; more broad-leaved 'Spica' (*L. latifolia*) is similar but grows to 'four Foot high'; and tuft-flowered 'Stoechas' (*L. stoechas*) is a 'shrub' growing 'three Foot high, the Leaves whitish Green and the Flowers a deep Purple' (Elizabeth Blackwell, *A Curious Herbal*, 1937–39).

❧ THE NAME The genus *Lavandula* is generally accepted as deriving from the Old French *lavandre* and the Latin *lavare* meaning 'to wash', referring to lavender's use in bathing, cleansing, perfume and to scent linen since Roman times. *Angustifolia* means 'narrow-leaved', *latifolia* 'broad-leaved', while *stoechas* stems from the Greek for 'in rows'. The Greeks also called lavender *nardus* after the Syrian city of Naarda where it was traditionally sold.

❧ THE PLACE Native to parts of the Mediterranean region, Africa, Asia and the Middle East, many species of lavender are now cultivated worldwide. All lavenders flourish best in light, free-draining, sandy or chalky soils in full sun. Drought-tolerant lavender also thrives in large terracotta or ceramic pots on a balcony or terrace and is ideal for coastal or gravel gardens.

❧ THE TIME Plant lavender in spring when the soil warms up and trim in late summer after flowering. Take non-flowering softwood cuttings in late spring or early summer, pot up when rooted and over-winter (protecting from frost) before planting out the following year. Harvest flowers when still in bud to help retain colour and fragrance.

❧ THE VIRTUES Used in ancient Egypt for embalming and cosmetics, by the Romans to dress war wounds, by the Persians to treat 'melancholia' (Avicenna, *Canon of Medicine*, 1025) and by Cleopatra as an alluring perfume, lavender has long been thought of as a cure-all. Lavender essential oil delivers the highest percentage of this herb's soothing, relaxing, antibacterial, anti-inflammatory and antiseptic properties.

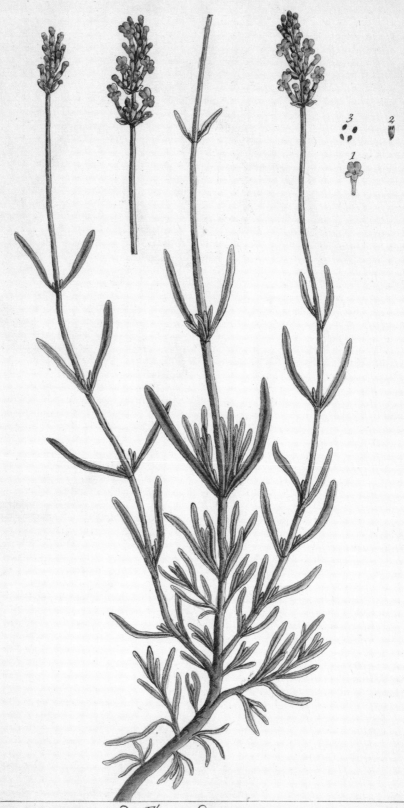

Plate 294.

Lavender.

1. Flower.
2. Cup.
3. Seed.

Lavendula.

Eliz Blackwell delin. sculp. et Pinx.

HEAL
LAVENDER HEALING SALVE

Use lavender salve to soothe insect bites
and small cuts, on temples to relax or
unwind, or as a moisturiser for dry face,
hands or body. You can also strengthen this
salve by using 250ml (1 cup) lavender-
infused oil (see page 18) in place of the
plain coconut oil.

Makes 10 x 28g (1fl oz) jars or non-reactive tins
**250ml (1 cup) organic fractionated coconut
oil, plus extra if needed**
**50g (1¾ oz) beeswax shavings or pellets, plus
extra if needed**
25 drops lavender essential oil

1 Place the beeswax in a heatproof bowl set
over a pan of simmering water or a double
boiler over a very low heat. Stir occasionally
until melted.

2 Add the coconut oil, stirring occasionally.
Add 25 drops of lavender oil.

3 Stir and check for a salve-like consistency
by spooning a little mixture into a spare
container and freezing for 2–3 minutes. Too
soft, add more beeswax; too firm, add more
coconut oil.

4 Remove from the heat. Pour the salve
mixture into non-reactive tins or jars. Set in
the fridge for around 10–15 minutes to
solidify. Add lids.

5 Use your fingers to apply where required.

Other uses
❧ Massage away aches and pains with a
soothing blend of sweet almond carrier oil
(250ml/1 cup) and 15 drops of lavender
essential oil.

❧ Decant a cooled lavender infusion
(see page 18) into a spray bottle to make
a calming spritz for face, body or home.

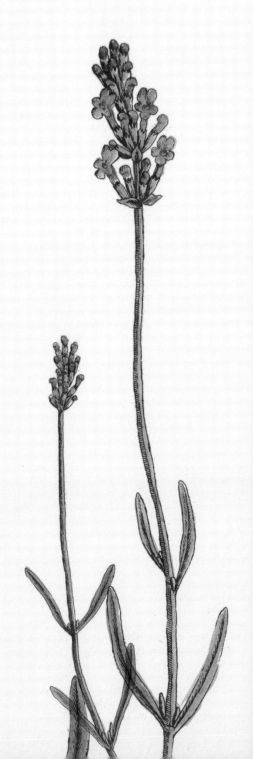

NOURISH
LAVENDER SUGAR

Most varieties of lavender can be used in cooking but those with the sweetest fragrance tend to work best. The most widely used 'culinary' lavender, *Lavandula angustifolia* 'Munstead', is ideal for making lavender sugar – a wonderful addition to shortbread, cakes and biscuits or stirred into summer berries.

Makes 1kg (2lb 4 oz)
1kg (5 cups) white caster sugar
2 tbsp dried or 4 tbsp fresh edible lavender flowers (in bud)

1 Place the sugar in a bowl.

2 Place a sieve over the bowl and push half the lavender through it. Mix the fine lavender powder into the sugar. Discard or compost what remains in the sieve.

3 Add the remaining lavender to the bowl and stir until evenly combined.

4 Pour the sugar into several sterilised, clip-top, glass storage jars – 10 x 100ml (3½fl oz) jars make lovely gifts, while 2 x 500ml (17½fl oz) jars are great for general storage.

5 Seal the jars and use as required. Lavender sugar will keep for up to a year.

Other uses
❧ Create an aromatic roasting rub using dried edible lavender buds, sea salt, black pepper, thyme and garlic powder.

❧ Simmer 250ml (1 cup) of runny honey with 2 tbsp of dried edible lavender to make the sweetest infused floral spread.

STYLE
LAVENDER DREAM PILLOW

Harness the soporific benefits of lavender by making a small 'pillowcase' filled with dried flower buds to use at night. Add a few drops of lavender essential oil for even sweeter dreams.

Makes 1 pillow
2 pieces of soft cotton fabric – 15cm x 7.5cm (6in x 3in) is ideal
500g (17½oz) dried lavender flower buds
Lavender essential oil to top up scent

1 Overlock or finish all edges of your fabric fto prevent fraying.

2 Place the fabric pieces right sides together and hand- or machine-stitch a 1.5cm (½in) seam around the edge. Leave an opening of 5cm (2in) on one short side.

3 Trim the corners to remove any bulk, press seams, turn out and press again.

4 Fill the pillowcase with lavender buds using a small funnel.

5 Top sew the opening closed, inserting a bespoke label if desired – ideal for gifts.

6 Use the pillow in bed or around the house wherever deep relaxation is required. To top up the scent, sprinkle 2–3 drops of lavender essential oil onto the pillow fabric.

Other uses
❧ Press aromatic, loosely arranged lavender sprigs into homemade beeswax candles before the wax sets for a nature-inspired decorative effect.

LOVAGE
Levisticum officinale, Apiaceae family

Elizabeth Blackwell's depiction of lovage pays equal homage to the root, stalks, leaves and seeds of this wonderfully versatile herb for good reason – all these plant parts have been documented as having medicinal and culinary purposes since at least Roman times. Although lovage seems to have fallen out of favour by the early twentieth century, given the advent of modern medicine and improved cultivation of its similarly tasting cousin celery, its strong parsley-celery-anise flavour and rustic charm has inspired a recent rebrand as a gourmet herb.

❧ **THE DESCRIPTION** Nicholas Culpeper sums lovage up in *The Complete Herbal* (1653) as a plant of 'large winged leaves, divided into many parts' and 'strong, hollow green stalks' growing to 'five or six, sometimes seven or eight feet hight' bearing 'large umbels of yellow flowers, and after them flat brownish seed'. The leaves, stem and seeds of lovage have a musky aroma and an intense, celery-like flavour.

❧ **THE NAME** Lovage's genus name *Levisticum* is thought to be a corruption of the earlier Latin *Ligusticum*, which refers to the Italian region of Liguria. While the common name lovage may derive from the word *levesche* – an Old French synonym for the plant – or from the Middle English *loveache*, 'ache' being an earlier word for lovage's cousin parsley.

❧ **THE PLACE** Dioscorides' *De Materia Medica* (AD 50–70) describes lovage as growing 'most plentifully in Liguria' where the inhabitants 'used it instead of pepper, mixing it with their sauces'. Thought to be native to western Asia as well as other parts of the Mediterranean, lovage requires moist but rich, well-drained soil, space and a sunny situation; it is a herb of 'easy culture' (Mrs M. Grieve, *A Modern Herbal*, 1931).

❧ **THE TIME** 'Lovage floureth most commonly in July and August', observes John Gerrard in his *Herball* (1597), while Elizabeth Blackwell notes it flowering 'in June' in A Curious Herbal (1737–39). To cultivate, sow seeds under cover in late summer and plant outdoors in early spring. Divide roots in spring or autumn.

❧ **THE VIRTUES** According to Nicholas Culpeper, lovage appears to be a cure for almost everything from 'spots and freckles' to 'the redness and dimness of the eyes'. Today this multi-tasking perennial has been revived as a warming addition to soups and stews, a component of confectionery and beverages, for its digestive and deodorising medicinal properties, and as a large garden ornamental.

Plate 275.

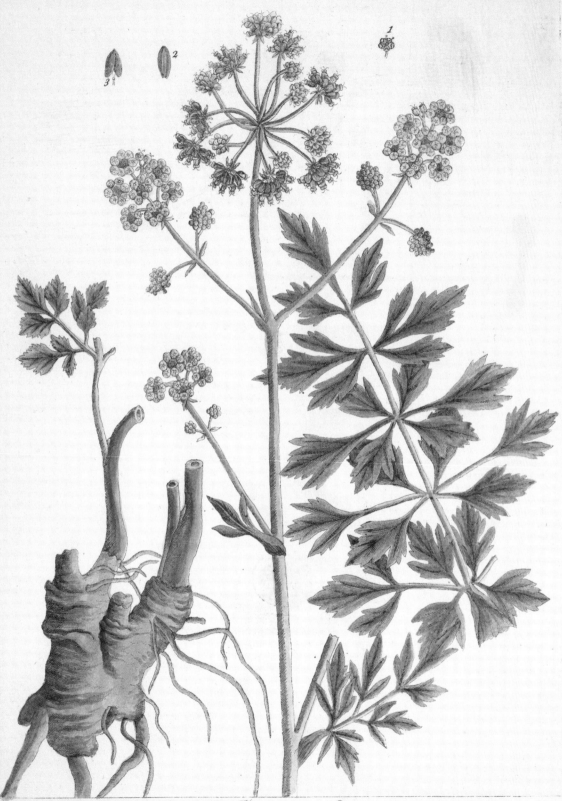

Lovage.

1. Flower.
2. Seeds.
3. The manner of
the Seeds Joyning.

Levisticum.

Eliz. Blackwell delin. sculp. et Pinx.

HEAL
SKIN-CALMING FOOT SOAK

According to folklore, medieval travellers used to stuff lovage leaves in their shoes to stay fresh and alert. Harness lovage's naturally deodorising properties today by adding to a therapeutic footbath at the end of a busy week.

Makes 1 foot soak
4 litres (4 quarts) warm (not boiling) water
Large handful of fresh or dried lovage leaves
8 drops lavender essential oil

1 Fill a large 5-litre (5-quart) foot-sized bowl with the water. Add the lovage leaves. Steep for 5 minutes.

2 Add the drops of the essential oil.

3 Place your feet in the bowl for at least 10 minutes to let tired soles soak up the herbal goodness.

Other uses
❧ Steep 1 tbsp of dried lovage leaves in 250ml (1 cup) of just-boiled water to make a restorative, digestive tea.
❧ Add a few drops of warming, spicy lovage essential oil to a home diffuser to calm the senses.

NOURISH
LOVAGE AND POTATO SOUP

Make nutritious lovage leaves the main ingredient in soups or salads; they work especially well with vegetables such as potatoes or peas. Small amounts of intensely flavoured lovage leaves or seeds used as a flavouring or garnish can go a long way, so be sparing.

Serves 4
2 tbsp butter
1 onion, chopped
1kg (2lb 4oz) potatoes, diced
750ml (3 cups) vegetable stock, plus extra if needed
500ml (2 cups) milk
4–5 handfuls of chopped fresh lovage leaves, plus extra to garnish
Salt and pepper to taste

1 Melt the butter in a large pan and sauté the onion. Remove from the pan, then sauté the potato. Add the onion back in and mix well.

2 Add the stock and milk and simmer until the potato is tender.

3 Remove from the heat, add the lovage leaves and puree with a hand blender. Add more stock if a thinner consistency is required.

4 Return to a simmer and season with salt and pepper.

5 Garnish with extra chopped lovage leaves and serve warm with other herby delights, such as rosemary focaccia (see page 120).

Other uses
❧ Harness the celery-parsley-aniseed flavour of lovage leaves or seeds to add an earthiness to stews.
❧ Use a hollow lovage stalk as a flavoursome straw in a Bloody Mary cocktail.

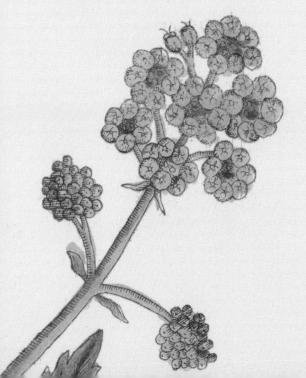

STYLE
CANDIED LOVAGE STEMS

Add a twist to a supper club, kids' party or festive table setting with jars of candied lovage stems to eat whole, use as sweet straws, or to decorate cakes. Replace lovage with angelica (see page 22) for a slightly different flavour.

Makes 10 stems
10 (approx. 500g/17½oz) fresh lovage stems
½ tsp bicarbonate of soda
Bowl of iced water
300g (1½ cups) granulated sugar

1 Peel the lovage stems and cut into even lengths to fit your selected storage jar.

2 Place in a pan, cover with 1.25 litres (5 cups) of water, add the bicarbonate of soda and boil for 5 minutes. Drain and then quickly plunge the stems into a bowl of iced water. Transfer to a clean glass bowl.

3 Combine 250ml (1 cup) water and 200g (1 cup) of the sugar in a pan. Boil into a syrup. Pour over the stems, covering with a cloth when the mixture reaches room temperature. Leave overnight.

4 Return the syrup to a pan, bring to a boil, add the stems and boil for 1–2 minutes.

Transfer the syrup and the stems to a bowl, bring to room temperature, cover and leave overnight again.

5 Repeat step 4 twice more, placing the stems on a rack to cool after the final boil.

6 Once the stems have dried, roll them in the remaining granulated sugar. Store in a jar or use as required. The syrup can also be used in soft drinks or cocktails.

Other uses
❧ Create beautiful botanical art by mounting pressed lovage flowers on a dark-coloured, velvety background.
❧ Turn leaves into a traditional syrupy cordial to add aniseed notes to brandy, Champagne or sparkling water.

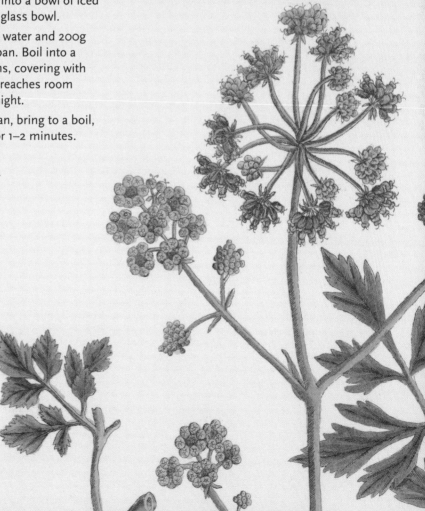

LEMON BALM

Melissa officinalis, Lamiaceae family

Lemon-scented and flavoured, leafy *Melissa officinalis* is an aromatic and potentially therapeutic addition to any herb garden or border. Persian physicians such as Avicenna were particularly effusive of lemon balm's virtues to help ease 'passions of the heart' and 'strengthen the vitall spirits' (John Parkinson, *Paradisi in Sole, Paradisus Terrestris*, 1629), whether they be 'rife from melancholy' or illness. Species of balm (*Melissa*) have also been much esteemed since ancient times for being particularly attractive to bees, thanks to the abundance of nectar in the flowers.

❧ THE DESCRIPTION Square-stemmed lemon balm 'grows 1 to 2 feet high, and has at each joint pairs of broadly ovate or heart-shaped, crenate or toothed leaves which emit a fragrant lemon odour when bruised. They also have a distinct lemon taste' writes Mrs M. Grieve (*A Modern Herbal*, 1931), plus 'white or yellowish' two-lipped flowers 'in loose, small bunches from the axils of the leaves'.

❧ THE NAME 'The word Balm is an abbreviation of Balsam, the chief of sweet-smelling oils', notes Mrs M. Grieve, while 'lemon' refers to its citrusy scent from the compounds citronellal, citral and geraniol. Lemon balm's genus name *Melissa* derives from the ancient Greek word for honey bee. Melissa was also a nymph who fed honey to the infant god Zeus in place of milk. *Officinalis* denotes a medicinal herb.

❧ THE PLACE Lemon balm is 'profitably planted in Gardens about places where Bees are kept' writes John Gerard in his *Herball* (1597), while Pliny suggests that 'bees find their way home by it'. Native to the Mediterranean, Iran and Central Asia, Gerard introduced lemon balm to his garden from Turkey, calling it 'Turky Balme'. Thanks to thousands of years of cultivation, the herb is now naturalised throughout Europe and North America.

❧ THE TIME Lemon balm is a hardy herbaceous perennial that can be cut back in summer to stimulate fresh new growth. It flowers between summer and autumn. Sow seeds indoors in spring and plant out after the first frost. Pick leaves throughout the summer for fresh use, plus freeze or dry batches of this fragrant herb (see page 16) to use year round for healing, cooking or beautifying.

❧ THE VIRTUES 'Hot and dry in the second degree' writes Avicenna (*Canon of Medicine*, 1025), lemon balm 'improves odour of the body ... is a tonic for the heart and also removes palpitations ... helps digestion and is useful in hiccough'. Now known to contain antioxidant, anti-inflammatory, antiviral and antimicrobial rosmarinic acid, lemon balm is useful in lip balms, skin tonics, digestive teas or to boost mood.

Plate 27.

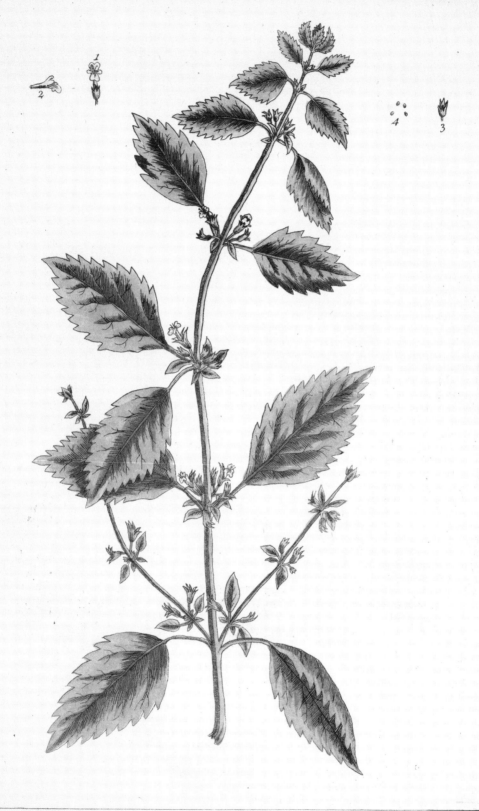

1 *Flower with its Cup*
2 *Flower Separate*
3 *Cup*
4 *Seed*

Melissophyllum

HEAL
BEE KIND LIP BALM

This gentle, antiviral and anti-inflammatory lip balm may help to speed up the healing time of cold sores and soothe minor cuts or dry skin.

Makes 6 x 30ml (1fl oz) non-reactive tins or pots
20ml (1½ tbsp) lemon-balm infused oil (made with olive oil or fractionated coconut oil – see simple preparations page 18), plus extra if needed
10g (1/3oz) beeswax (shaved or pellets), plus extra if needed
120g (½ cup) shea butter
10 drops lemon balm essential oil
4 drops peppermint essential oil (optional)
2 drops tea tree essential oil (optional)

1 Combine the oil, beeswax and shea butter in a double boiler or a glass bowl over a pan of boiling water. Heat gently until everything has melted.

2 Check for a lip-balm-like consistency by spooning a little mixture into a spare container and freezing for 2–3 minutes.

Too soft, add more beeswax; too firm, add more lemon-balm infused oil.

3 Remove from the heat, add the lemon balm essential oil, plus peppermint and tea tree essential oils if desired. Stir gently.

4 Pour the mixture into small non-reactive tins or jars and place in the fridge for 10–15 minutes to set. Add lids. Use daily on sore or chapped lips or skin.

Other uses
❧ Add a few drops of lemon balm essential oil to an aromatherapy diffuser to help lift mood and inspire joy.
❧ Crush fresh lemon balm leaves and rub onto exposed skin to help keep irritating mosquitoes at bay.

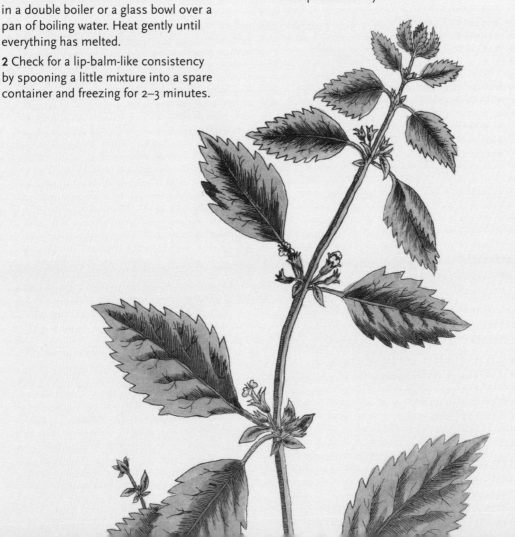

NOURISH
LEMON BALM ICED TEA

'John Hussey of Sydenham, who lived to the age of 116, breakfasted for fifty years on Balm tea sweetened with honey,' writes Mrs M. Grieve in *A Modern Herbal* (1931). Also said to help reduce fever, soothe the nerves, cheer the heart and refresh the mind, lemon balm tea might just be the perfect antidote for our modern times.

Serves 4
2 litres (2 quarts) cold water
Large handful of fresh lemon balm leaves, washed, plus extra to garnish
4 tbsp raw honey
20 ice cubes
4 slices of lemon or lime

1 Bring the water to a boil in a large pan.

2 Add the lemon balm leaves and honey. Remove from the heat, cover and steep for 30 minutes.

3 Strain out the leaves and allow the tea infusion to cool.

4 Place 5 ice cubes each in four 450ml (16fl oz) glass jar 'mugs'. Fill almost to the brim with lemon balm tea.

5 Garnish each with fresh lemon balm leaves and a slice of lemon or lime.

Other uses
❦ Freeze fresh lemon balm leaves for later use in teas or as an infusion for ice cream.
❦ Tear washed fresh lemon balm leaves into hot, buttered peas or broad beans for a spring-fresh side dish.

STYLE
LEMON BALM BOUQUET

Lemon balm foliage is verdant from spring through to autumn and holds its own in a vase of water making it ideal for flower arrangements. Its leafy stems, wildflower blooms and lemon-scented leaves also add an uplifting fragrance to any bouquet.

Makes 1 bouquet/vase or several jam jars
Large bunch of fresh lemon balm stems, ideally with flowers
Selection of seasonal herbs or flowers such as lavender, fennel, dahlias or roses

1 Gather a bunch of lemon balm stems from the top of the plant to help promote bushier growth. Trim stem ends and place in water.

2 Gather 3–5 stems each of contrasting blooms. Trim the ends.

3 Strip leaves from the bottom of all stems and arrange naturalistically in a bouquet or large vase. Keep turning for a balanced arrangement. Or cut stems shorter and place in a selection of jam jars.

4 Place around the house to scent as well as beautify, or use as a centrepiece for a herb-inspired dinner.

Other uses
❦ Use lemon balm infused oil to create antiviral and naturally exfoliating, olive-green soap bars for home use, guests and gifts.
❦ Create a summery perfume by combining lemon balm (5 drops), lavender (1 drop) and rose absolute (4 drops) essential oils in 2 tsp of sweet almond carrier oil. Mix in a rollerball bottle and apply to wrists, neck and elbows.

MINT
Mentha, Lamiaceae family

The distinctively scented garden stalwart, mint, has been one of the world's best-known culinary, medicinal and cosmetic herbs since antiquity. More than 20 variously flavoured and beneficial species including spearmint/garden mint (*Mentha spicata*), corn mint (*M. arvensis*), horse/wild mint (*M. longifolia*), water mint (*M. aquatica*), bergamot/orange mint (*M. citrata*), apple/pineapple mint (*M. suaveolens*) and pennyroyal (*M. pulegium*) plus well-known medicinal hybrids such as peppermint (*M. × piperita*) grow wild and are cultivated all over the world.

❧ THE DESCRIPTION From the '20 remedies' of 'wild mint' or '*mentastrum*' of Pliny (*Naturalis Historia*, AD 77–79) to the comprehensive roll-call found in Mrs M. Grieve's *A Modern Herbal* (1931), there's no doubt that members of this genus are prolific cross-breeders. Top of most lists are the sweeter-tasting spearmint and the intensely menthol-flavoured peppermint. Both have fuzzy, toothed leaves and tiny, pale purple-lilac flowers.

❧ THE NAME Although mint is noted as *Eduosmos*, *Emeros* or *Eduosmos Agrios* in Dioscoride's *De Materia Medica* (AD 50–70), he also alludes to the Egyptian name *tis* and the Roman word *menta*, root of the genus *Mentha*. This is thought to reference an ancient Greek myth concerning the nymph Minthe (also Menthe, Mintha or Mentha) who was transformed into a sweet-smelling plant by Zeus's daughter Persephone.

❧ THE PLACE This hugely cosmopolitan herb is fine in shade or full sun but does prefer reliably moist, well-drained soil. Peppermint, a hybrid of watermint and spearmint, has its native range in Europe and Central Asia, spearmint's origins extend from Europe to China, while horsemint/wild mint's roots stretch across Europe, Asia, the Middle East and Africa. In gardens, contain mint in a pot to restrict its invasive roots.

❧ THE TIME Pick fresh mint leaves through spring and summer or harvest for drying in late summer when 'the plants are breaking into bloom ... on a dry day, after the dew has disappeared, and before the hot sun has taken any oil from the leaves' (*A Modern Herbal*, 1931). Hang loose bunches of mint to dry then rub through a fine sieve into a jar to store. Propagate by dividing and potting up sections of root in autumn.

❧ THE VIRTUES Mint's many applications are described in great detail in Nicholas Culpeper's *Complete Herbal* (1653) and include preventing milk curdling, treating dog bites and as a digestive. Spearmint contains carvone, thought to settle the stomach, while menthol-rich peppermint is prized both as a soothing tea and a versatile essential oil. That minty flavour and aroma also lends itself to a range of culinary and cosmetic uses from pea and mint soup to toothpaste.

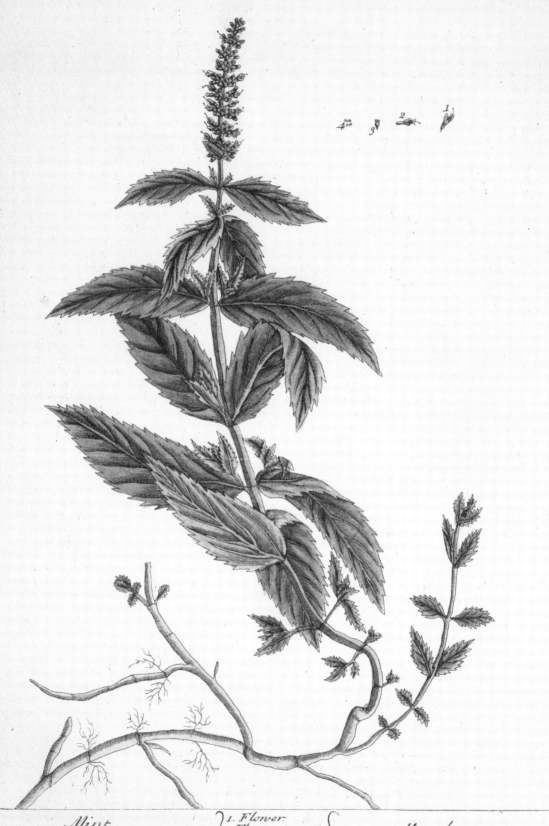

Plate 290.

Mint.

1. *Flower.*
2. *Flower separate.*
3. *Calix.*
4. *Seed.*

Mentha.

Eliz. Blackwell delin. sculp. et Pinx.

HEAL
MOROCCAN MINT TEA

Mint tea is synonymous with Morocco, where it has supposedly been sipped since the 12th century BC, as a sacred ritual drink as well as a refreshing beverage traditionally offered to guests and visitors. The tea is rich in antioxidants and menthol that can help boost the immune system and ease congestion.

Makes 6 servings

1 tbsp Chinese gunpowder green tea
1.25 litres (1¼ quarts) just-boiled water
3–4 tbsp sugar or 3–4 sugar cubes
Large handful of fresh mint leaves, plus
**   extra sprigs to garnish**

1 Place the tea in a large (1 litre/1 quart) Moroccan teapot with strainer included.

2 Pour in 250ml (1 cup) of the water and swirl gently to warm the pot, rinsing the tea at the same time. Strain out the water but keep the leaves.

3 Add the remaining water to the teapot. Steep for 2 minutes.

4 Stir in the sugar and add the torn mint leaves. Steep for a further 3–4 minutes.

5 Serve in Moroccan tea glasses, pouring from a forearm's height to help create a foamy 'head'. Add a sprig of fresh mint to garnish and serve immediately.

Other uses
❁ Combine coconut oil, baking powder, stevia powder (sweetener) and peppermint essential oil to make naturally minty toothpaste.
❁ Dilute 2–3 drops of peppermint essential oil in 1 tbsp of fractionated coconut oil – rub on the neck and temples to help soothe a headache.

NOURISH
PEA AND MINT SOUP

Celebrate summer by serving this classic combination of fresh peas and mint. The peas add sweet, delicate notes and a refreshing gorgeous green colour, while the mint adds zing.

Serves 2

Large handful of fresh mint leaves
1 onion
1 garlic clove
1 tbsp olive oil
600g (4 cups) fresh petit pois
500ml (2 cups) vegetable stock
2 tbsp crème fraîche, to serve
Fresh pea shoots to garnish

1 To make mint-leaf ice cubes, place a few small mint leaves in water in an ice-cube tray. Freeze overnight or until set.

2 Finely chop the onion. Crush the garlic. Gently fry both in the oil until translucent.

3 Stir in the petit pois and vegetable stock and simmer for around 5 minutes.

4 Let mixture cool slightly. Tear in the mint leaves. Whizz with a stick blender until smooth and even.

5 Serve the soup chilled in small bowls or enamel mugs with mint-leaf ice cubes, a dollop of crème fraîche and a garnish of pea shoots.

Other uses
❁ Chop fresh mint and cucumber into creamy yogurt to make a cooling *raita* dip for popadums or spicy curries.
❁ Mix fresh mint, salt, sugar, water and vinegar to make a traditional sweet-tangy mint sauce for roasts.

STYLE
CLASSIC MOJITO

This traditional Cuban highball, one of the most refreshing and stylish cocktails for a hot summer day, may have started as a 16th-century remedy for scurvy, made from ingredients sourced around Havana by sailors in Sir Francis Drake's fleet. Fresh lime could certainly have eased the ailment, while mint and sugarcane juice would have helped disguise the harshness of the rum.

Serves 1
1 lime
Saucer of kosher salt, sea salt or granulated sugar (to garnish glass rims)
10 fresh mint leaves, plus a sprig to garnish
1 tbsp granulated sugar
Crushed ice
50ml (2oz) white rum
Splash of soda water

1 Quarter the lime and use one quarter to wet the rim of a highball glass. Lightly roll the rim in kosher salt, sea salt or granulated sugar.

2 Place two lime wedges in the glass along with the mint leaves and sugar. Muddle with a spoon to release the lime juice and bruise the mint.

3 Add a layer of crushed ice to almost one third of the way up. Pour over the rum.

4 Add a splash of soda water to taste, stir with a long spoon, garnish with a fresh mint sprig and the last wedge of lime.

Other uses
❧ Use orange mint, chocolate mint or pineapple mint as garnishes and invite friends to taste the difference.
❧ Blend peppermint extract with sugar, chocolate, butter and Golden syrup to make a delicious batch of peppermint patties.

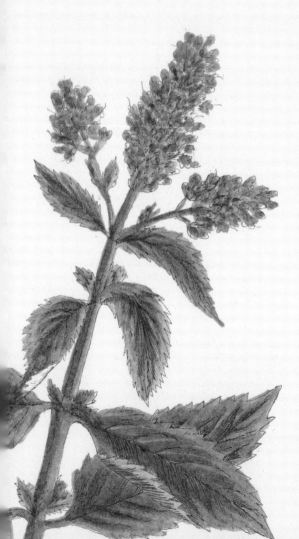

Peppermint, *Mentha* × *piperita*.

SWEET CICELY
Myrrhis odorata, Apiaceae family

One of two accepted species in the same family as parsley, *Myrrhis* is among the lesser known culinary and medicinal herbs. All parts of this strongly aniseed-scented perennial are edible: feathery grass-green leaves, creamy-white umbels, brown-black elongated fruits and even the root. Traditionally used to treat stomach ailments, coughs and bruises, as a blood purifier, natural wood polisher, salad ingredient and a natural sweetener for tart fruit such as rhubarb and gooseberries, it was also grown by Carthusian monks in the 18th century as one of the main ingredients of the liqueur Chartreuse.

❧ THE DESCRIPTION Sweet cicely (*Myrrhis odorata*) is so similar in looks to other umbellifers such as cow parsley (*Anthriscus sylvestris*) and toxic hemlock (*Conium maculatum*) that correct identification is vital. All have hollow stems, creamy-white umbels, fern-like leaves and parsnip-like taproots, but sweet cicely has more delicate, downier, anise-scented leaves, smaller flowers and longer seeds that turn black when ripe. Consult a guide if unsure or grow your own.

❧ THE NAME Mrs M. Grieve lists numerous common names for sweet cicely in *A Modern Herbal* (1931) including British myrrh, anise, sweet chervil, smooth cicely, sweet-fern and shepherd's needle. The genus name *Myrrhis* derives from the ancient Greek word for an aromatic oil from Asia, while *odorata* means 'scented'. Cicely stems from the ancient Greek word *seselis*, traditionally used to describe a range of umbelliferous plants.

❧ THE PLACE Thought to be native to central and Mediterranean Europe, including Albania, Austria, France, Germany, Italy, Spain and Switzerland, sweet cicely has also been widely introduced and naturalised throughout the verges, woodlands, grasslands and riverbanks of Scandinavia, the UK, Poland, and parts of Central Europe and Russia. Grow in moderately fertile, moist but well-drained soil in dappled shade.

❧ THE TIME This prolific perennial provides a ready crop of sugary, anise-tasting leaves and stems through spring, summer and autumn. Leaves taste sweetest before flowering, which occurs in mid-spring to early summer, followed by the spicy, edible seeds in autumn. The large, thick taproot can also be dug up and eaten, and is at its most nutritious in late autumn. Propagate by seed sown outdoors when ripe.

❧ THE VIRTUES 'This plant is often eat as a Sallad, being much of the same Nature as Chervil consisting of hot and thin Parts being good for cold windy Stomachs', reads Elizabeth Blackwell's still relevant description of sweet cicely (*A Curious Herbal*, 1737–39). Sweet cicely is now known to be antioxidant, high in vitamins, minerals and beta carotene, although its most widespread use is as a natural sweetener for fruit puddings, pies and compotes.

Plate 243.

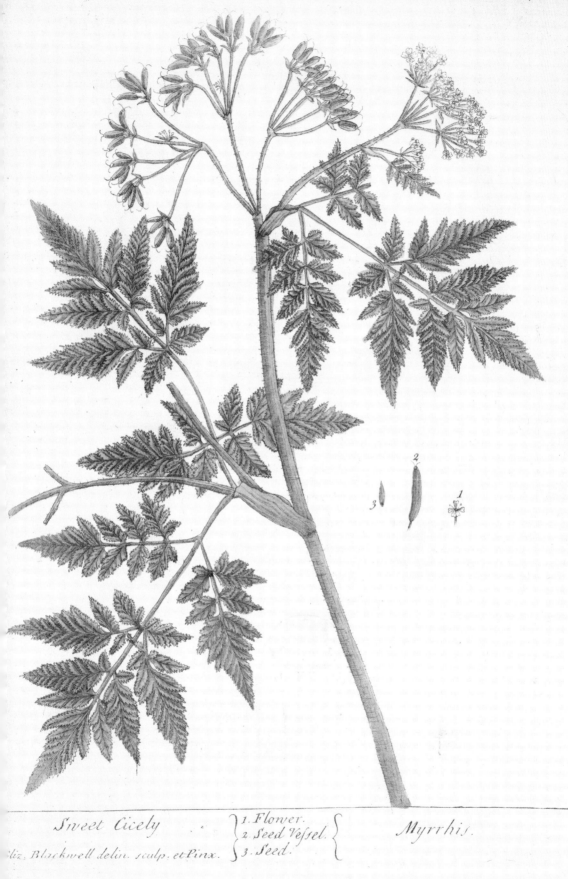

Sweet Cicely
1. Flower.
2. Seed Vessel.
3. Seed.
Myrrhis.

Eliz. Blackwell delin. sculp. et Pinx.

HEAL SWEET CICELY KOMBUCHA

Combine the carminative properties and anise flavour of sweet cicely with the antioxidant, potentially gut-healing benefits of kombucha in this tangy fizzy drink.

Makes 1 x 1 litre (1 quart) bottle
Small bunch of sweet cicely (stems and leaves)
200g (1 cup) granulated sugar
1 tbsp black or green loose-leaf tea
1 kombucha SCOBY (mother)

1 Wash the sweet cicely. Place the black or green tea in a tea infuser or ball.

2 Boil 1 litre (1 quart) water in a large pan. Remove from the heat. Add the tea, sweet cicely and sugar. Leave to infuse for 5 minutes. Stir occasionally to mix.

3 Remove the tea infuser or ball. Leave to cool. Strain the liquid through muslin into a sterilised 4 litre (1 gallon) lidded jar.

4 Add the kombucha mother to the strained liquid. Cover the jar with muslin. Place in a cool, dry place for 2 weeks.

5 Remove the kombucha mother from the jar. Reserve for the next batch by storing in a jar of kombucha liquid, in the fridge.

6 Strain the remaining liquid through muslin into a sterilised 1 litre (1 quart) airtight bottle. Seal. Store in the fridge for 3 months. Consume within 10 days of opening, starting with a few sips to get used to the flavour and effects.

Other uses
❧ Infuse 2–3 tsp of dried ground sweet cicely root in 250ml (1 cup) of just-boiled water for a wind-relieving tea.
❧ Chew on ripe sweet cicely seeds to freshen breath or as sugar-free sweeties.

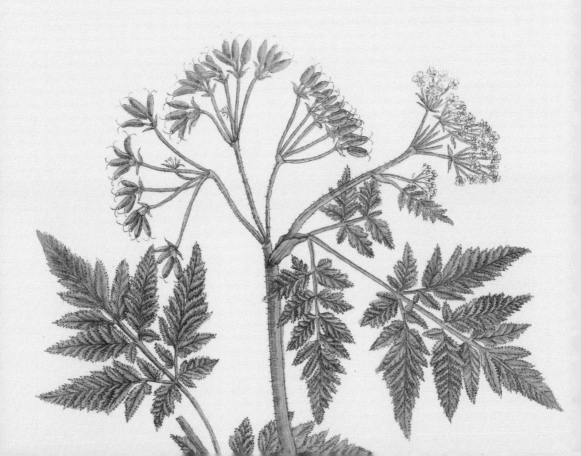

NOURISH SWEET CICELY AND RHUBARB COMPOTE

The subtle anise flavour of sweet cicely is an ideal foil for tart fruits such as rhubarb or gooseberries. Throw a handful into the stew pot when preparing fruit for crumble, combine with ginger in a tangy-sweet compote, stir into yogurt, or spread on waffles or French toast.

Makes 2 x 250ml (8fl oz) jars
4 large rhubarb stems (around 400g/14oz)
Large bunch of sweet cicely (leaves and stems)
2.5cm (1in) cube fresh ginger
2 tbsp granulated sugar or honey

1 Wash the rhubarb and chop into 2.5cm (1in) chunks. Wash the sweet cicely and chop finely. Peel and grate the ginger.

2 Place all the ingredients in a large pan. Cook for around 10 minutes on a low heat. Stir continuously until the rhubarb softens. Add 1 tbsp of water if required.

3 Remove from the heat. Leave to cool slightly. Decant the finished compote into two sterilised airtight 250ml (8fl oz) glass jars.

4 Seal with lids and store in a fridge for up to 2 weeks. Or freeze in batches in an ice-cube tray.

Other uses
❧ Infuse milk with sweet cicely leaves to make a pale-green, slightly liquorice-flavoured custard to pour over fruit or puddings.
❧ Sweet cicely is also great in savoury dishes such as salads, soups, béarnaise sauce, roasted root vegetables or tempura.

STYLE SWEET CICELY SCHNAPPS

This sweet, spicy, highly aromatic, green-golden schnapps tastes a little like Greek *ouzo* or French *pastis*. The leaves, stems, flowers or seeds of the plant impart a delicate liquorice-anise flavour into the vodka. Drink as an aperitif or digestive shot, pour over ice for a neat drink, or use as a base for a cocktail.

Makes 1 x 1 litre (1 quart) bottle
Large bunch of sweet cicely stems, leaves, flowers and seeds
100g (½ cup) granulated sugar
750ml (3 cups) vodka

1 Harvest and wash the sweet cicely.

2 Place in a sterilised airtight 1 litre (1 quart) glass jar with the sugar.

3 Pour the vodka over, seal and shake to mix.

4 Leave to infuse in a cool dark place for 2–3 weeks. Agitate every few days.

5 Decant into another sterilised airtight 1 litre (1 quart) glass bottle and discard the herbs. Seal and store in a cool dark place.

Other uses
❧ Use lightly crushed, unripe green seeds and leaves of sweet cicely as a traditional furniture polish – simply wipe over untreated wooden surfaces such as oak.
❧ Plant lacy sweet cicely for contrast alongside robust rhubarb crowns – both emerge in early spring and make the perfect culinary pairing.

BASIL

Ocimum basilicum, Lamiaceae family

This tender, aromatic herb of 'love washed with tears', as immortalised in John Keats' poem *Isabella, or The Pot of Basil* (1818), has been celebrated and feared in equal measure with varied attributes including a harbinger of misfortune, a tyrannical breeder of scorpions and a cure for their bites, a homage to the dead, and a Renaissance-era dating advertisement. Where pots of sweet basil (*Ocimum basilicum*) or bush basil (*Ocimum minimum*) were once placed on windowsills to signify romance, they are now tended for their culinary potential.

❧ **THE DESCRIPTION** Sweet basil (*Ocimum basilicum*) has 'one upright stalk, diversely branching forth on all sides, with two leaves at every joint, which are somewhat broad and round, yet pointed, of a pale green colour, but fresh, a little illipt about the edges, and of a strong heady scent. The flowers are small and white, flowering at the tops of the branches, with two final leaves at the joints' (Nicholas Culpeper, *Complete Herbal*, 1653).

❧ **THE NAME** The genus name *Ocimum* is an ancient Greek name for the basil plant, possibly derived from the word *ozo* 'to smell'. The species name *basilicum* comes from the ancient Greek word *basilikós* and the Latin *basilicum* for 'royal'. These kingly or queenly associations explain why the French sometimes refer to sweet or garden basil as '*l'herbe royale*'.

❧ **THE PLACE** Various *Ocimum* species are native to many tropical parts of Asia, Africa and America, but have been widely cultivated in the Middle East and Europe for centuries. Flourishing best in warmer climes and a rich soil, they include sweet or garden basil (*Ocimum basilicum*), 'Thai Basil' (*O. basilicum* var. *thyrsiflora*), bush basil (*O. minimum*), lemon basil (*O.* × *citriodorum*) and holy basil (*O. tenuiflorum*).

❧ **THE TIME** Basil 'must be sowed late, and flowers in the heat of the summer, being a very tender plant', advises Culpeper in his *Complete Herbal* (1653). While Mrs M. Grieve in *A Modern Herbal* (1931) advises sowing seeds in a 'hotbed' (greenhouse or indoors) in early spring, then moving to a warm border in early summer. It is ideal for a container in a sunny spot. Pluck leaves as required, which also encourages new growth to appear.

❧ **THE VIRTUES** Astrologer-herbalist Nicholas Culpeper considers basil a 'herb of Mars' and 'under the Scorpion', declaring it good for bee stings and expelling the afterbirth. By the 1930s, upon publication of *A Modern Herbal* (1931), 'aromatic' and 'carminative' (wind-relieving) basil is a fully-fledged culinary and medicinal herb. It is now known to be high in antioxidants, with antibacterial and anti-inflammatory properties.

Plate 104.

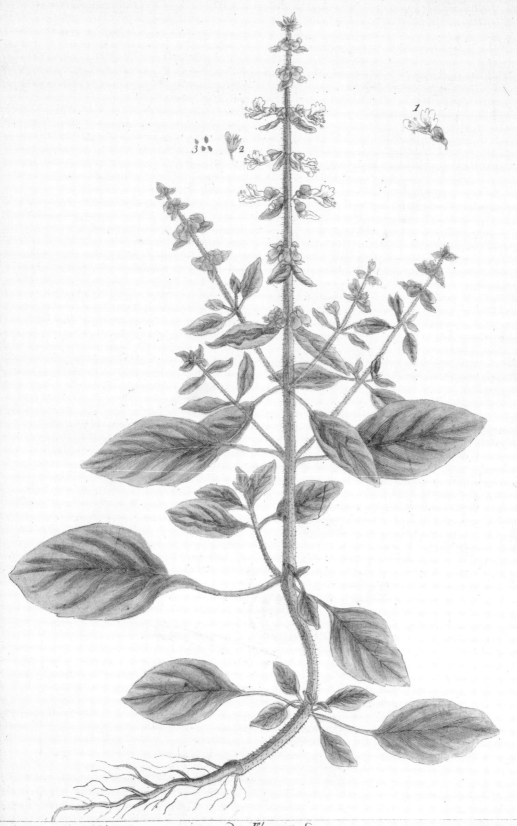

Basil

liz. Blackwell delin. sculp. et Pinx.

1. *Flower*
2. *Fruit*
3. *Seed*

Basilicon or Ocimum.

HEAL
HEAD-EASING STEAM

Harness basil's anti-inflammatory properties to help get rid of tension headaches, best administered via a relaxing steam inhalation. Or for relief on the go, try chewing on a few fresh basil leaves.

Makes 1 inhalation
500ml (2 cups) hot water
1 tbsp dried basil leaf

1 Pour the water into a large bowl and add the basil – you can use shop bought basil or dehydrate your own by hanging bundles of 15cm (6in) stems upside down in a dark, warm, dry place, or by drying single leaves on a low setting in a dehydrator.

2 Place a towel over your head and the bowl. Then carefully inhale the steam for 10–15 minutes until your headache begins to subside.

Other uses
❧ Sip on hot basil and honey tea or gargle a cooled basil infusion to help soothe a sore throat.
❧ Place a few drops of basil essential oil on clothing to help aid concentration.

NOURISH PESTO ALLA GENOVESE

Originating in Genoa, Italy, the recipe for this famous basil sauce was first published in the gastronomic *La Cuciniera Genovese* (1863). The word pesto hails from the Italian word *pestare* meaning 'to pound'. For the silkiest texture, pound with a pestle and mortar, rather than blitz in a blender.

Makes 1 x 250ml (8fl oz) jar
Large bunch fresh basil leaves
2 garlic cloves
2 tbsp pine nuts
¼ tsp fine sea salt
125ml (½ cup) extra virgin olive oil, plus extra to cover
25g (¼ cup) finely grated Parmesan
50g (½ cup) finely grated Pecorino

1 Remove the stems from the basil leaves. Peel and bruise the garlic cloves.

2 Grind the leaves, pine nuts, garlic and salt into a rough paste using a pestle and mortar or a blender.

3 Pour in the olive oil, continuing to pound until evenly mixed. Mix in the finely grated Parmesan and Pecorino cheeses.

4 Transfer to an airtight 250ml (8fl oz) jar, then cover with a thin layer of olive oil.

5 Stir the pesto into pasta, dot on pizza, use as a marinade or smudge onto bread.

Other uses
❧ Prepare an heirloom Caprese salad of heritage tomatoes, mozzarella, torn basil leaves, balsamic vinegar and olive oil.
❧ Basil pairs well with strawberries, citrus fruits, watermelon, peanut butter and chocolate, so experiment with puddings or desserts.

STYLE SWEET BASIL FLOWER OIL

When a basil plant flowers it begins to put its energy into making seeds rather than leaves. The usual advice is to pinch off blossoms as soon as they appear, although the pretty purple-white, albeit milder-tasting flowers are edible too. Use them as a garnish for canapés or drinks, or to create a pretty bottle of infused oil.

Makes 1 x 350ml (12fl oz) bottle
Handful of fresh basil flowers (washed)
375ml (1½ cups) extra virgin olive oil
Few sprigs of dried basil flowers (optional)

1 Place the fresh basil flowers in a sterilized, airtight 350ml (12fl oz) glass bottle or oil dispenser.
2 Cover the flowers with the oil and seal tightly with a lid or a stopper.
3 Place the jar on a sunny windowsill for at least 4 hours – ideally 24 hours – to infuse.
4 Remove the fresh flowers to avoid mould. Replace with dried basil flower sprigs for decorative effect, if desired.
5 Drizzle over salad, pasta or pizza or use in dressings. This infused oil also looks super pretty on a table alongside a similar vessel of balsamic or herb-infused vinegar.

Other uses
❧ Explore different species of basil. 'Dark Opal' basil (*Ocimum basilicum* var. *purpureum*) also looks great in a bouquet or vase.
❧ Muddle together a 'gin basil smash' cocktail of basil leaves, lemon juice, sugar syrup, gin and ice.

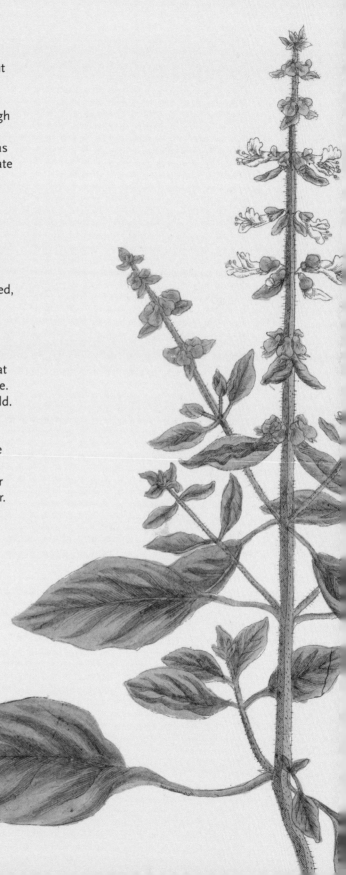

MARJORAM
Origanum majorana, Lamiaceae family

Also known as sweet marjoram or knotted marjoram, this creeping, white or pinkish flowered, velvety-leaved plant shares many of the same physical features as well as part of its name with wild marjoram or oregano (*Origanum vulgare*, see page 106). Where the two plants differ most is in the taste and aroma; marjoram is sweet, floral and 'woodsy', whereas oregano is pungent, citrusy and camphorous. Marjoram has also been used for centuries as a soothing sleep aid and a warming perfume note.

❧ THE DESCRIPTION John Gerard and Nicholas Culpeper refer to 'sweet marjoram' (*Origanum majorana*) alongside 'pot marjoram' (*O. onites*) and 'winter marjoram' (*O. vulgare* var. *hirtum*), now known as Greek oregano. All look similar, with a creeping habit and small, round leaves but sweet marjoram generally has paler leaves and knots of white or pinkish flowers. If in doubt, taste it for sweetness.

❧ THE NAME Dioscorides refers to marjoram in *De Materia Medica* (AD 50–70) by its ancient Greek name *Sampsuchon* but also notes *Amaracum* (Sicilian), *Sopho* (Egyptian) and *Majorana* (Roman) – the latter leading to marjoram's common and species name. The genus name *Origanum* is thought to stem from the Greek words *oros* (mountain) and *ganos* (brightness) alluding to oregano's native habitat (see page 106).

❧ THE PLACE Originating in Cyprus and Turkey, marjoram was introduced to a wide range of countries including Greece, the UK, Italy, Morocco, Spain, Switzerland and India. Grow in containers (for easy moving) in a sunny, sheltered spot in soil with added grit.

❧ THE TIME Sow marjoram seeds indoors in early spring, planting out in early summer when all danger of frost has passed. Marjoram hates to sit in cold, damp soil so avoid overwatering and move plants into a sheltered spot or indoors in winter. The flowers bloom in late summer, with the most flavoursome leaves picked just before the flower buds open.

❧ THE VIRTUES 'Indeed, sir, she was the sweet Marjoram of the salad, or rather, the herb of grace', said the Clown in Act IV, Scene V of William Shakespeare's *All's Well That Ends Well* (1623), alluding to marjoram's reputation as a 'herb of joy'. Warming, comforting marjoram is still a very popular culinary herb and the essential oil can soothe muscles or aid relaxation.

Plate 319.

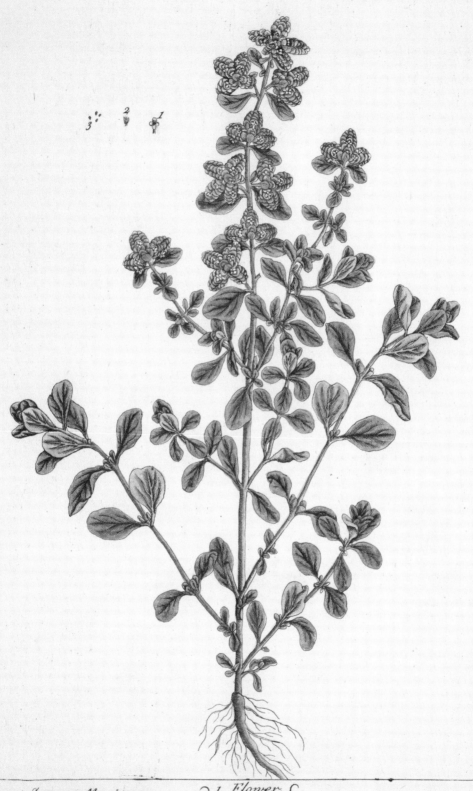

Sweet Marjoram. $\Big\{$ 1. *Flower.* $\Big\{$
3

2

1

$\Big\{$ 2. *Cup.* $\Big\}$ *Majorana.*

Eliz. Blackwell delin. sculp. et Pinx.   3. *Seed.*

HEAL MUSCLE RELIEF
MASSAGE OIL

Combine the sweet scent and warming, muscle-relaxant properties of sweet marjoram essential oil with nourishing sweet almond oil to create a deeply therapeutic massage oil for tired bodies, aching joints or poor circulation. Add a few drops of lavender essential oil for deeper relaxation and rosemary essential oil for extra pain relief.

Makes 1 x 50ml (1¾fl oz) bottle
3 tbsp sweet almond oil
10 drops sweet marjoram essential oil
10 drops lavender essential oil
7 drops rosemary essential oil

1 Almost-fill a 50ml (1¾fl oz) brown- or blue-tinted and capped bottle with the sweet almond carrier oil.

2 Add the essential oils using a dropper.

3 Close the bottle with a lid and shake gently to mix.

4 Massage oil into areas of muscle or joint pain, or use for a therapeutic full body treatment – perfect after a warm shower or bath.

Other uses
❧ Fill a rollerball bottle with 10ml (1/3fl oz) sweet almond oil and 2 drops of sweet marjoram essential oil for a soothing, sensory pick-me-up.
❧ Add ¼ tsp of dried marjoram leaves and flowers, a stick of lemongrass and 1 tsp of honey to 250ml (1 cup) of just-boiled water for a vitamin- and mineral-rich tea.

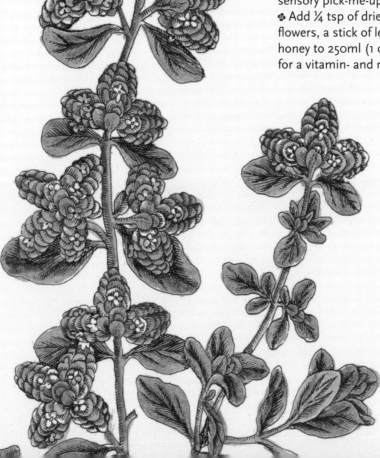

NOURISH
ZA'ATAR SPICE MIX

Za'atar refers not only to marjoram's close relative Syrian oregano (*Origanum syriacum*) – the herb most likely to be the 'hyssop' mentioned in the Bible (see page 70) – but also to a popular Middle Eastern mix of herbs and spices. Traditional ingredients are sweet marjoram, oregano, thyme and sumac (made from the dried fruits of Sicilian sumac or *Rhus coriaria*) mixed with sesame seeds and salt.

Makes 1 x 180ml (6fl oz) jar
1 tbsp sesame oil
1 tbsp sesame seeds
4 tbsp sumac
2 tbsp fresh thyme
2 tbsp dried marjoram
2 tbsp dried oregano
1 tsp sea salt flakes

1 Warm the sesame oil in a pan and lightly toast the sesame seeds until golden.

2 Combine the seeds with the rest of the ingredients and grind in a pestle and mortar. Transfer to a 180ml (6fl oz) jar.

3 Keep in the fridge for up to 3 months. Offer a dish of *za'atar* alongside a dish of olive oil as a tangy herby dip for pitta bread, use in marinades or rubs, or sprinkle onto yogurt, stews, soups or pizza.

Other uses
❧ Add fresh marjoram at the last moment of cooking to introduce a mild, sweet, Mediterranean flavour to roast vegetables, cheese, eggs, beans or mushrooms.
❧ Marinate tofu overnight in a mix of balsamic vinegar, crushed garlic, marjoram and salt.

STYLE SLEEP-EASY
LINEN SPRAY

Scent bed linen, pillows or even pyjamas with a spray of sleep-easy sweet marjoram and relaxing lavender. Store in an elegant blue or amber glass bottle to protect the oils from light and keep it by the bedside or give to a sleep-deprived loved one.

Makes 1 x 500ml (17½fl oz) spray bottle
500ml (2 cups) distilled water
1 tbsp bicarbonate of soda
15 drops sweet marjoram essential oil
15 drops lavender essential oil

1 Place the water in a 500ml (17½fl oz) tinted-glass spray bottle.

2 Add the bicarbonate of soda and the essential oils and swirl gently to mix – use a wooden stick to stir if necessary.

3 Seal the bottle with a spray top and cap.

4 Spritz a little linen spray on sheets, pillows or nightwear at bedtime to help beat insomnia or promote a peaceful night's sleep.

Other uses
❧ Grow marjoram in between vegetables to help deter greenfly and blackfly.
❧ Combine a few drops each of sweet marjoram and lemongrass essential oils with pink Himalayan bath salts to create a relaxing, restorative bath soak.

OREGANO
Origanum vulgare, Lamiaceae family

Strongly aromatic oregano (*Origanum vulgare*) is often confused with sweet marjoram (*Origanum majorana* – see page 102), not only on account of its common name of wild marjoram but also owing to its similarly oval leaves, square stems and whorled flower spikes. Oregano's scent and flavour is much more pungent, camphorous and bitter, however, and the flowers a deeper, pinky purple, sweeping many a native mountainside with joyful colour. A favoured culinary, medicinal and fragrancing herb of ancient Greece and Rome, dried oregano remains synonymous with Greek and Italian cuisine.

❀ **THE DESCRIPTION** 'Wild or Field Marjoram', notes Nicholas Culpeper (*A Complete Herbal*, 1653), 'has a root which creeps much under ground' and 'brownish, hard, square stalks with small dark green leaves, very like those of sweet Marjoram, but harder, and somewhat broader; at the top of the stalks stand tufts of flowers, of a deep purplish red colour. The seed is small, and something blacker than that of sweet Marjoram.'

❀ **THE NAME** John Gerard's 'wilde Marjerome', Nicholas Culpeper's 'Common Wild Marjoram' or '*Origanum vulgaris*', Dioscoride's '*Agrioriganos*' and Pliny's '*Heracleotic Origanum*' are all types of *O. vulgare* (Linnaeus, 1753). The genus name stems from the Greek words *oros* for 'mountain' and *ganos* for 'brightness', in homage to the 'herb of joy' in its native habitat. *Vulgare* denotes a commonly found plant.

❀ **THE PLACE** Oregano is native to a wide swathe of Europe, the Middle East, Central Asia and North Africa and naturalised in parts of North and South America. Subspecies include the culinary favourite *Origanum vulgare* subsp. *hirtum* or Greek oregano. In Britain, look for oregano (*Origanum vulgare*) on dry, infertile, alkaline soils in habitats such as chalk or limestone grassland, hedge banks or woodlands. Grow in a warm sunny position.

❀ **THE TIME** Surface-sow fine oregano seeds indoors in spring, planting out in early summer when all risk of frost has passed. Avoid over-watering. Harvest in late summer, picking leaves before the flower buds open to use fresh – or tie in loose bunches and store in a warm, well-ventilated space to dry. Bring plants indoors in winter for a year-round supply of flavoursome and medicinal leaves.

❀ **THE VIRTUES** Elizabeth Blackwell (*A Curious Herbal*, 1737–39) recommends oregano for 'Obstructions of the Liver Breast & Womb; helping the Jaundice, shortness of Breath & stoppage of the Menses' as well as for headaches and toothache. Today, oregano is best known as a common ingredient of pizza sauce and pasta, as well as a potent antibacterial, antifungal, antioxidant and potentially pain-relieving essential oil.

Plate 280.

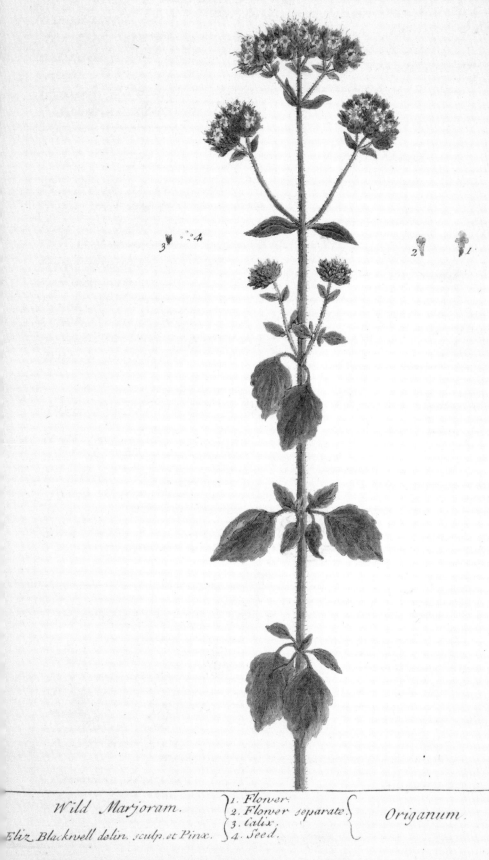

Wild Marjoram.

1. Flower.
2. Flower separate.
3. Calix.
4. Seed.

Origanum.

Eliz. Blackwell delin. sculp. et Pinx.

HEAL
HAPPY FEET OIL

Oregano essential oil contains a powerful combination of antioxidants and phenols including carvacrol, thymol and rosmarinic acid – traditionally harnessed to help fight bacterial and fungal infections of the feet such as athlete's foot. Combine with apple cider vinegar, sweet almond oil and warm water for a medicinal foot soak, or prepare the therapeutic oil below to massage directly into skin or nails.

Makes 1 x 10ml (1/3fl oz) dropper bottle
2tsp fractionated (liquid) coconut oil
8 drops oregano essential oil

1 Almost-fill a 10ml (1/3fl oz) amber-coloured glass dropper bottle with the coconut oil.

2 Add the drops of oregano essential oil. Seal with the dropper lid.

3 Massage the oil into the affected area of skin or nails three times a day. Put on a clean sock to help stop the oil from rubbing off.

Other uses
❧ Sip on an infusion of fresh or dried oregano leaves and honey steeped in boiling water to help soothe a sore throat or cough.
❧ Massage oregano essential oil diluted in sweet almond carrier oil into the lower back and stomach to aid digestion.

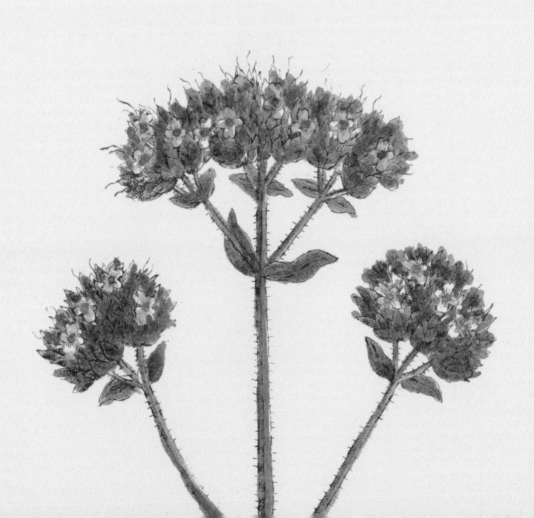

NOURISH
AROMATIC PIZZA SAUCE

Oregano adds a tangy note to pizza sauce alongside the sweeter taste of basil (see page 98). Fresh oregano is more pungent than dried oregano so measure accordingly.

Serves 4–6
10 fresh tomatoes (or 2 x 400g/14oz tins, chopped)
1 onion
3 tbsp extra virgin olive oil
3 large garlic cloves, crushed
2 tbsp red wine vinegar
Small handful of fresh basil or 1 tsp dried
Small handful of fresh oregano or 1 tsp dried
2 tbsp tomato purée
Pinch of sugar
Salt and black pepper to taste

1 Dice the tomatoes and onion.

2 Heat the oil in a large pan and cook the onion until golden. Lower the heat, add the garlic and then the red wine vinegar. Simmer gently for 1–2 minutes.

3 Add the tomatoes, basil and oregano and simmer for 20 minutes (5 minutes for tinned tomatoes). Stir occasionally.

4 Add the purée, sugar and salt and pepper to taste. Simmer for 5 minutes. Remove from the heat. Whizz with a stick blender until smooth.

5 Store in the fridge in sterilised, airtight jars for 1 week, or freeze for 2 months.

6 Spread onto pizza dough using the back of a spoon, or use as a pasta sauce.

Other uses
❖ Sprinkle fresh oregano leaves, a little garlic, chilli, Parmesan and olive oil onto pasta for a taste of the Mediterranean.
❖ Drizzle fresh oregano pesto over smoky baked aubergine served with caramelised red onion and toasted pine nuts.

STYLE
HERB OF JOY CAKE

Spread some happiness with this moist, zesty, herbaceous Italian-inspired ode to the ancient 'herb of joy'.

Makes 1 cake
butter, for greasing
2 oranges
2 lemons
150g (¾ cup) granulated sugar
4 eggs
2 tbsp dried oregano
100ml (1/3 cup) olive oil
120g (1 cup) plain flour, plus extra for dusting
50g (½ cup) almond flour
1 tsp baking powder
500g (4 cups) icing sugar
Small handful of fresh oregano leaves

1 Preheat the oven to 180°C (350°F). Grease and lightly flour a 23cm (9in) non-stick Bundt or spring-form cake tin with butter. Zest and juice the oranges and lemons.

2 Beat the sugar, eggs and half the lemon and orange zest together until creamy.

3 Add the dried oregano and then drizzle in the oil. Beat until well mixed.

4 Sift the flours and baking powder into the bowl. Gently fold in.

5 Pour the mix into the prepared cake tin and bake for around 40–45 minutes. Turn out onto a rack and leave to cool.

6 Combine the remaining orange and lemon zest, all of the juice and the icing sugar to make a glaze. Drizzle over the top of the cake. Decorate with tiny sprigs of fresh oregano.

Other uses
❖ Dry bunches of purple-pink oregano flowers to use in pot pourri or dried flower bouquets.
❖ Add a fresh oregano sprig to a classic Negroni of gin, vermouth and Campari.

PARSLEY
Petroselinum crispum, Apiaceae family

Fresh-tasting, curly parsley leaves are easily dismissed as a retro garnish, but this underestimates just how powerful a herb parsley is. Native to just a very small area of the Balkans, its ubiquity as a plant of 'universal esteem', as referenced in Pliny's *Naturalis Historia* (AD 77–79), stems from widespread cultivation since ancient times. It is not, however, just the green parts of the plant that have been traditionally used but also the seeds and roots. Benefits include flavouring, freshening and easing the digestion of foods, plus less palatable links to Greek funeral rites and the devil.

❧ THE DESCRIPTION Cultivated forms of flat-leaf French and Italian parsley (*Petroselinum crispum* 'French' and *P. crispum* var. *neopolitanum*) appear similar to wild or species parsley (*P. crispum*), although the latter's leaves have curlier edges. The bushy biennial plants bear rich green, 1–3-pinnate leaves (year one) and umbels of small, yellow-green flowers (year two). Other cultivated forms include parsnip-rooted Hamburg parsley (*P.* var. *tuberosum*) and others with very tightly curled leaves.

❧ THE NAME Ancient parsley synonyms date back to Theophrastus, the word *selinon* being key. *Oreoselinon* or *Petroselinon* (rock selinon) refer to parsley, and evolved into the Latinised genus name *Petroselinum* and the common name parsley, while *Heleioselinon* or *Eleioselinon* (marsh selinon) refer to celery (*Apium graveolens*). *Crispum* means 'curly' and is also confusingly applied to flat-leaved parsley.

❧ THE PLACE When cultivated forms of parsley spread across Europe, Central and South East Asia, South and Central America and parts of northern and South Africa, so the herb became incorporated into local cuisines and medicinal folklore. To grow, choose a site with deep, fertile but well-drained soil in sun (but out of midday sun) or partial shade.

❧ THE TIME Broadcast or drill-sow parsley seeds outdoors in beds or pots from late spring to the start of summer, renewing plants every two years. Mrs M. Grieve (*A Modern Herbal*, 1931) advises sowing three times in late winter and mid-spring for a good summer harvest, and mid-to-late summer to overwinter in a cold frame. Harvest fresh leaves year-round, drying in loose bunches or freezing to prolong use.

❧ THE VIRTUES Parsley is now known to be a rich source of the antioxidant compound chlorophyll, the green pigment in plants, plus it's packed with vitamins and minerals such as vitamins A, B, C and K, and iron and potassium. Parsley is a natural cleanser and diuretic but also stimulates menstruation so avoid taking as a tea, tincture or eating large amounts during pregnancy.

Plate 172.

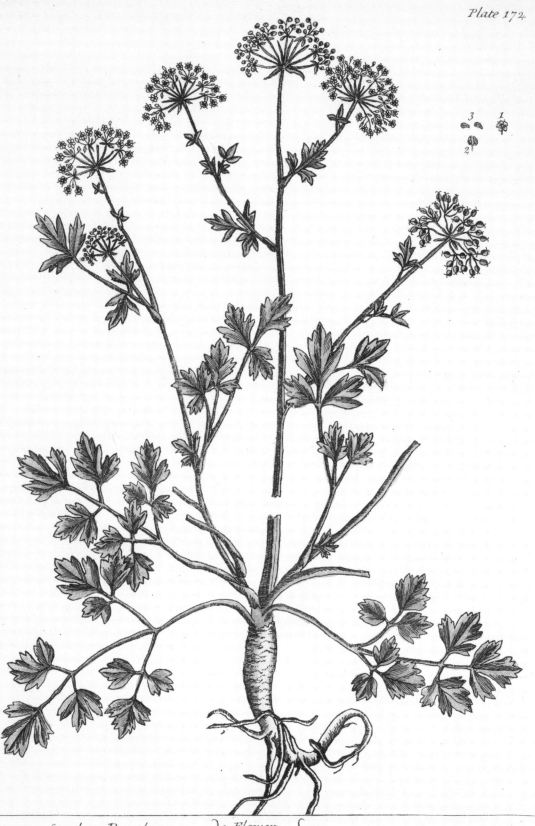

Garden Parsley

Eliz. Blackwell delin. sculp. et Pinx.

1. Flower.
2. Seed Vessel.
3. Seed.

Apium hortense or Petroselinum.

HEAL
PARSLEY DETOX JUICE

Parsley is the ideal ingredient for a detoxifying green juice. Blend a bunch with 250ml (1 cup) just-boiled water and the juice of a lemon, or combine with other health-boosting ingredients such as spinach, apple, cucumber or celery to provide the nutritious and cleansing all-in-one boost below (juicer required).

Serves 2
2.5cm (1in) cube fresh ginger
1 lemon
1 green apple
½ cucumber
1 stick celery
Large bunch of parsley (leaves and stems)
2 large handfuls of baby spinach leaves

1 Peel and halve the ginger. Remove the peel and pith from the lemon and chop into quarters. Chop the apple, cucumber and celery in pieces to fit through a juicer.

2 Set 2 of the lemon quarters aside. Feed all the other ingredients into the juicer. Alternate between leaves and harder elements to help push things through.

3 The resulting juice should be a lovely bright green. Check for taste and if desired, squeeze in the remaining lemon wedges. Serve immediately.

Other uses
❧ Drink a tea of fresh parsley leaves steeped in 250ml (1 cup) just-boiled water to help combat water retention. Avoid during pregnancy.
❧ Chew fresh parsley to help alleviate bad breath. Dip leaves in a little apple cider vinegar first to potentially increase effectiveness.

NOURISH
TABBOULLEH

Traditional Middle Eastern tabboulleh – served as a refreshing main or side – is all about the parsley, which is mixed with bulgur wheat, chopped mint, fresh tomatoes, lemon juice and olive oil. Add Lebanese spice or fruits to personalise.

Serves 2–4
100g (½ cup) bulgur wheat
250ml (1 cup) just-boiled water
4 bunches of flat-leaf parsley
1 bunch of garden mint
5 medium tomatoes
5cm (2in) piece of cucumber
1 shallot or 3 spring onions
3 tbsp olive oil
1 tsp flaked sea salt
Juice of 1 lemon
1 tsp *baharat* or Lebanese seven-spice mix
90g (½ cup) pomegranate seeds

1 Rinse the bulgur wheat until the water runs clear. Drain well, transfer to a bowl and pour in the just-boiled water. Cover, soak for 20 minutes, then drain.

2 Wash the parsley and mint in very cold water. Remove the stems and slice both herbs finely being careful not to bruise. Pat dry.

3 Dice the tomatoes and strain to remove some of juice. Peel and dice the cucumber. Finely slice the shallot or spring onions. Place in a large bowl together.

4 Add the bulgur wheat, herbs, olive oil, salt, lemon juice, *baharat* or Lebanese seven-spice mix and pomegranate seeds. Mix well and serve.

Other uses
❧ Flavour soup or stew with a classic *bouquet garni* of fresh or dried parsley, thyme and bay.
❧ Cook a handful of chopped parsley into a herby Middle Eastern omelette.

STYLE CHIMICHURRI GREEN SAUCE

This incredibly versatile Argentinian parsley-garlic-chilli sauce is lovely drizzled over canapés or entrées for a party. It also pairs well with avocados, eggs, potatoes or tofu, although the classic combination is steak. Make a big bowl for guests to pass around *asado* (Argentinian barbecue) style.

Makes 1 sharing bowl
2 bunches of fresh parsley
Bunch of coriander leaves (optional)
2 sprigs of oregano (optional)
2 spring onions
2 garlic cloves
1 tbsp crushed chilli flakes or 1 red jalapeño, chopped
4 tbsp apple cider vinegar
Juice of 1 lemon
250ml (1 cup) extra virgin olive oil
Flaked sea salt and black pepper to taste

1 Remove the parsley stems. Roughly chop the leaves. Repeat for the coriander and oregano, if using.

2 Finely slice the spring onions. Peel and finely mince the garlic. Place together with the herbs in a large mortar or a blender.

3 Add the chilli flakes or red jalapeño, apple cider vinegar, lemon juice, olive oil, and salt and pepper to taste.

4 Use a pestle to mix the ingredients and bruise the herbs, or blitz briefly in a blender.

5 Cover and chill for 3 hours or overnight to fully macerate. Serve as desired.

Other uses
❧ Grow curly parsley as an ornamental edging around other herbs, or any parsley as a flavour-enhancing, pest-repelling companion for roses, tomatoes or carrots.
❧ Replace classic mint with the slightly peppery taste of parsley in a gin julep cocktail muddled with fresh lime.

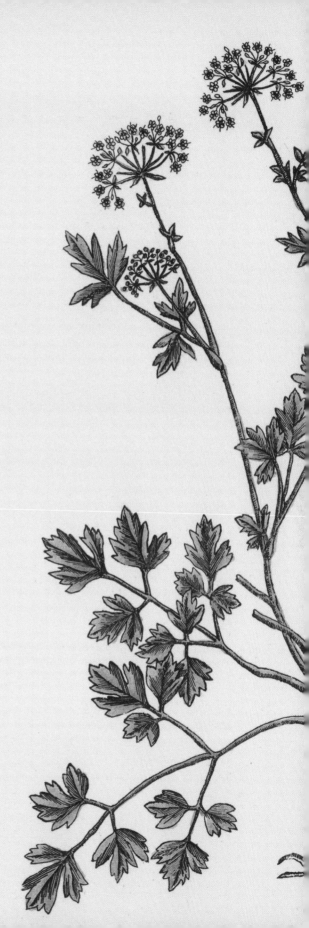

ROSE
Rosa, Rosaceae family

'What a pother have authors made with Roses! What a racket have they kept?' exclaimed Nicholas Culpeper (*Complete Herbal*, 1653) in tribute to one of the most highly prized plants in herbal history. From the unctuous *oleum rosaceum* (infused rose oil) of Dioscorides' *De Materia Medica* (AD 50–70), through Middle Eastern preparations for rose water and rose otto (steam-distilled rose oil), to the numerous teas, tinctures, infusions, balms and culinary uses described in today's herbals, the rose's reputation for healing, beautifying and imbuing with exquisite taste is richly deserved.

❧ THE DESCRIPTION Species roses are woody perennials with five-petal flowers, sharp prickles and pinnate leaves. Millennia of hybridisation and cultivation, however, has led to numerous forms including white *Rosa alba*, red *R. gallica*, dog rose (*R. canina*), sweet briar rose (*R. rubiginosa*), deeply fragrant damask rose (*Rosa* × *damascena* – pictured) and Provence or cabbage rose (*Rosa* × *centifolia*).

❧ THE NAME The ancient Greek philosopher and 'Father of botany' Theophrastus refers to cultivated roses as *Rhodon* (red), from which the genus name *Rosa* and plant family name Rosaceae evolved. Species names for roses are wonderfully evocative from *Rosa canina* (dog rose), thought to allude to a cure for the bite of a mad dog to *Rosa* × *damascena* (damask rose) from supposed origins around Damascus, Syria.

❧ THE PLACE At least 150 species roses are native to and can still be found wild in temperate parts of Asia (*R. chinensis*; *R. banksiae*; *R. rugosa*), Europe (*R. canina*; *R. gallica*; *R. arvensis*; *R. rubiginosa*; *R. spinosissima*; *R. villosa*), North America (*R. gymnocarpa*) and the Middle East (*R.* × *damascena*). For the best blooms, give cultivated roses at least six hours of direct sunlight and rich soil.

❧ THE TIME Elizabeth Blackwell's *A Curious Herbal* (1737–39) cites the damask, white and red roses as flowering in varying months of summer. Some species roses also flower in spring and others will keep blooming into autumn. Harvest petals or buds after the dew has dried but before midday for the strongest scent. Remaining flowers turn into red or orange, vitamin C-rich hips, becoming softer, fleshier and most useful in autumn after the first frost.

❧ THE VIRTUES From ancient Greek eyelid-easing ointments (Dioscorides, *De Materia Medica*, AD 50–70) to tales of Roman excess where roses were seemingly strewn everywhere (Mrs M. Grieve, *A Modern Herbal*, 1931), this gorgeous 'herb' has long been valued for its fragrance, astringent properties (particularly *R. gallica*) and perfumed flavour (*R.* × *damascena*). Roses are also beautiful in any garden, table setting or bouquet.

Plate 82.

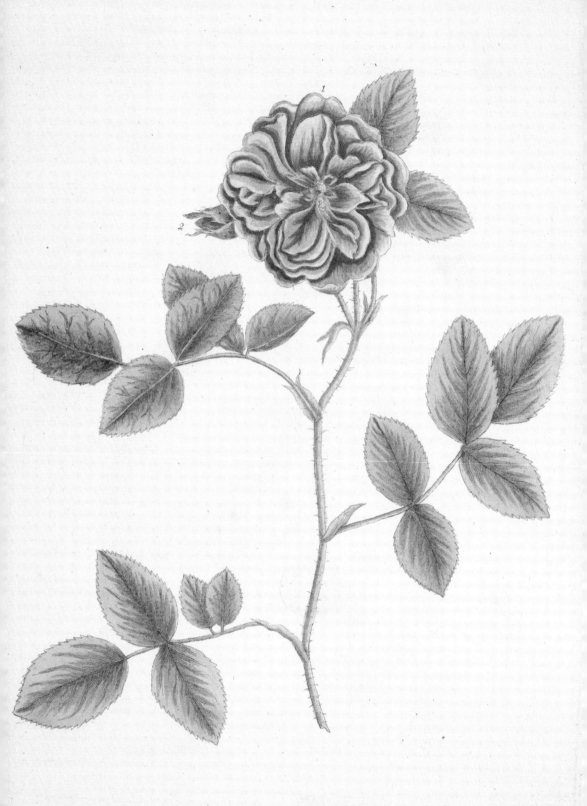

The Damask Rose

Eliz. Blackwell delin. sculp. et Pinx.

1. Flower
2. Bud

Rosa Damascena

HEAL
ROSE WATER HYDROSOL

For the sweetest-scented, beautifying, therapeutic or even edible rose water, make a steam-distilled hydrosol in place of a simple infusion, garnering a few drops of rose essential oil in the process.

Makes 1 x 500ml (17½fl oz) hydrosol
5–6 handfuls of fresh or dried, red or pink scented rosebuds – damask rosebuds are ideal
1.5 litres (1½ quarts) distilled water
Ice (preferably in sealed bags)
Rose essential oil (optional)

1 Use pesticide-free, almost-open rosebuds from the garden or hedgerow, or source dried from a store. Remove the stamens, sepals and white sections if necessary.

2 Place a ceramic ramekin upside down in the centre of a large, glass-lidded pan. Add the rosebuds and distilled water until level with the ramekin. Do not over-fill.

3 Stand a bowl on the ramekin. Cover the pan with an upside-down lid. Heap ice (in bags for easy placement) on top of the lid.

4 Heat on low until the petals look spent and the rose hydrosol has collected in the bowl. Replace ice as necessary.

5 Remove the pan from the heat and let the captured hydrosol cool. Carefully decant into a sterilised 500ml (17½fl oz) sterilised, tinted-glass jar or spray bottle.

6 Store in a cool, dark place and use as required. For additional scent and medicinal benefits, add a few drops of rose essential oil.

Other uses
❀ Make a replenishing face oil of rosehip and avocado oil, plus rose essential oil.

❀ Calm nerves or lift spirits with a daily tonic of sweet-tasting, homemade rose glycerite (rose petals infused in glycerine).

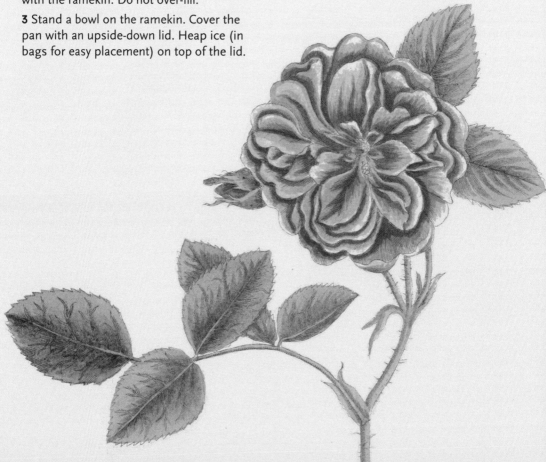

NOURISH
ROSE HIP SYRUP

Vitamin C-rich rosehips lend themselves to jellies, sauces, soups, seasonings and tea, but rosehip syrup, usually made with dog rose (*R. canina*) fruits, is the most traditional and quite delicious.

Makes 2 x 250ml (8 fl oz) bottles
1kg (2lb 4oz) topped and tailed ripe rosehips – use dog rose (*R. canina*) or Japanese rose (*R. rugosa*)
250g (1 cup) sugar or 175g (½ cup) raw honey

1 Wash the hips, then mince in a blender. Place in a pan with around 1.5 litres (1½ quarts) of water or enough to cover. Bring to a boil, turn off the heat and set aside for 15 minutes.

2 Strain the resulting rob (condensed juice) through a muslin cloth into a jug. Strain again until all irritant hairs have been removed. Compost the hip remnants.

3 Place the rob in a clean pan, bring to a boil and then simmer again until reduced to around 500ml (17½fl oz). Add the sugar or honey. Simmer until syrupy and leave to cool slightly.

4 Decant into hot 250ml (8fl oz) sterilised airtight glass bottles leaving a 1cm (½in) gap at the top. Seal with a bung.

5 Store in the fridge unopened for 3 months, opened for 3–4 weeks. Take 10ml (2 tsp) of immune-boosting syrup once or twice a day or add 15ml (1 tbsp) to 250ml (1 cup) of just-boiled water for a warming drink.

Other uses
❦ Use rose-petal-infused honey as a fragrant sweetener for teas or yogurt, or as a treat on its own.

❦ Combine rosewater with cardamoms, pistachios, or oranges for Persian-inspired confectionery or cakes.

STYLE CRYSTALLISED
ROSE PETALS

Take inspiration from Mrs M. Grieve's 'Recipe for Crystalized Roses' in *A Modern Herbal* (1931) to create attractive decorations for cakes, desserts or drinks. Adapt this recipe for other edible flowers too.

Makes 20–30 crystallised petals
Selection of petals from organically grown roses
1 egg white, lightly beaten
50g (¼ cup) caster or 50g (½ cup) icing sugar

1 Collect rose petals on a dry, sunny day when flowers are fully open. For edible petals, roses must be pesticide- and pollution-free. Remove bugs.

2 Place the egg white in one saucer and the sugar in another. Use tweezers to dip petals into the egg and then the sugar. Use a small paintbrush to get the mixture into folds.

3 Shake off any excess sugar. Leave the petals on baking parchment in a warm, dry place for 24–48 hours until fully dry.

4 Store between parchment sheets in an airtight container. Use as desired.

Other uses
❦ Shower brides and grooms with fresh or dried rose-petal confetti given to guests in hand-rolled paper cones.

❦ Arrange single stems or bouquets of highly fragrant roses around the house for their beauty and to lift your spirits.

ROSEMARY
Rosmarinus officinalis, Lamiaceae family

Needle-leafed and blue-flowered, this evergreen shrub is one of the easiest herbs to identify because its foliage has a strong, distinctive taste and a camphorous, balsamic odour. 'The Ancients were well acquainted with the shrub, which had a reputation for strengthening the memory', notes Mrs M. Grieve in *A Modern Herbal* (1931), further describing rosemary as an emblem of 'fidelity for lovers' and a 'herb for magical spells' and 'religious ceremonies' that was also used to 'purify the air and prevent infection'. A reliable culinary ingredient, many a roast has been improved with just a few sprigs.

❧ THE DESCRIPTION Both wild and cultivated rosemary have a woody framework with branching stems, linear leaves with felty undersides, two-lipped flowers born in small clusters and a pungent aroma of pine. The flowers vary from deep to pale blue, to white or pale pink, and forms may be upright or prostrate (creeping); the latter is ideal for trailing over walls.

❧ THE NAME *Rosmarinus* stems from the Latin words *ros* and *marinus* or 'dew of the sea', in reference to rosemary's native habitat of coastal dry scrub and rocky hillside. Synonyms include the ancient Greek *Libanotis* (Dioscorides, *De Materia Medica*, AD 50–70) and Pliny, *Naturalis Historia* (AD 77–79), denoting an incense-scented herb. *Libanotis coronaria* specifically alludes to rosemary's use in crowns.

❧ THE PLACE Although native to warmer regions of the Mediterranean such as Spain, Greece, Italy, Egypt and Turkey plus parts of northern Africa, rosemary is also reasonably hardy in colder climes. Plant in the garden or grow in pots in poor, well-drained soil in a sunny, fairly sheltered position, avoiding ground that stays wet over winter.

❧ THE TIME Rosemary is easy to cultivate, best started in the spring from ready-grown plants or propagated from semi-ripe cuttings in spring or late summer. Germination from seed is slow and not always successful. To ensure a plentiful supply of young, succulent stems for culinary use, gather leaves regularly and prune each spring. Rosemary leaves and flowers can also be dried or frozen for later use.

❧ THE VIRTUES The many and varied traditional uses of rosemary include: a 'remedy against the fluffing of the head' (John Gerard, *Herball*, 1597); in bath oils and ointments to warm the joints; as a stimulating hair tonic; and a nerve-calming wine or tea. Rosemary is now known to include rosmarinic acid, which brings antioxidant, anti-inflammatory, anti-fungal and stimulating benefits. It is also delicious in food.

Plate 159.

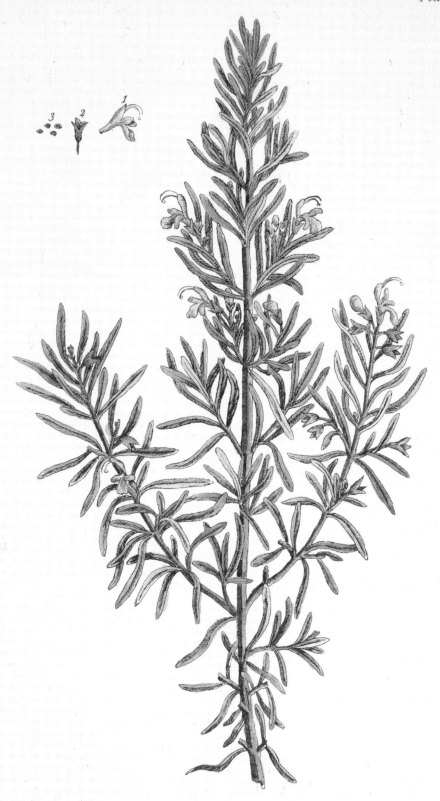

HEAL INVIGORATING HAIR RINSE

Rosemary makes a naturally stimulating rinse to boost circulation, promote glossier and thicker hair, or help treat an itchy scalp. Breathe in the woody, floral scent as the rinse works its therapeutic magic.

Makes 1 x 500ml (17½fl oz) spray bottle
6 sprigs of fresh rosemary

1 Bring 500ml (2 cups) of water to a boil in a small pan.

2 Strip the rosemary leaves from the stems and drop into the water. Reduce the heat, cover (to stop volatile oils escaping) and gently simmer for 2–3 minutes. The solution should turn a dark brown with an oily surface film.

3 Allow the liquid to cool and then strain into a 500ml (17½fl oz) sterilised glass mister bottle, closing with a spray cap. Compost the discarded rosemary.

4 Spritz onto hair after shampooing, massaging in until all the liquid has been absorbed. Leave on hair for at least 20 minutes.

5 Rinse with cool water to help close the cuticle on the hair shaft and bring added shine. Comb gently and allow hair to dry.

Other uses
❧ Sip on rosemary tea, containing the compound carnosic acid, to help promote healthy gut bacteria and nutrient absorption.
❧ Combine 2 drops of rosemary essential oil with 10ml (1/3oz) sweet almond oil to make a circulation-boosting, skin-smoothing massage oil.

NOURISH ROSEMARY FOCACCIA

Bake a batch of traditional Italian *focaccia di Genova* complete with salt, olive oil and aromatic sprigs of rosemary.

Makes 1 loaf
135ml (4½fl oz) olive oil, plus extra for oiling
6 sprigs of fresh rosemary
300g (2½ cups) strong white bread flour
7g (1/8oz) fast-action yeast
2 tsp flaked sea salt
175ml (¾ cup) tepid boiled water

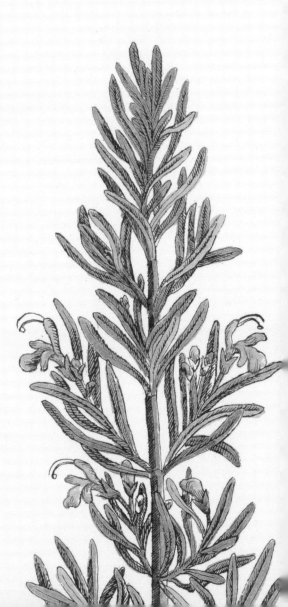

1 Infuse 6 tbsp of the olive oil with 4 sprigs of rosemary in a bowl for 30 minutes. Decant the oil into a drizzler.

2 Combine the flour, yeast, remaining olive oil and 1 tsp of the sea salt in a separate bowl. Slowly add the tepid water to make a sticky dough.

3 Knead the dough on a lightly oiled surface until elastic. Place in a lightly oiled bowl. Cover with a cloth. Leave for 1 hour.

4 Preheat the oven to 200°C (400°F). Gently knead the dough again. Place on a lightly oiled baking sheet. Shape into a loose rectangle measuring about 20 x 28cm (8 x 11in).

5 Indent the dough at regular 4cm (1½in) intervals with a floured finger. Break off smaller pieces from the remaining rosemary sprigs and push into each hole. Allow the dough to rise for another 30 minutes.

6 Sprinkle with the remaining sea salt, drizzle with two thirds of the rosemary-infused olive oil and bake for 25–30 minutes until well risen and pale golden brown.

7 Remove from the oven. Drizzle with the remaining oil. Serve immediately or cover.

Other uses
❧ Make an aromatic roasting rub by infusing sea salt with lemon zest and rosemary sprigs.
❧ Rosemary also works well paired with peaches, lemons, fennel, grapefruit or chocolate.

STYLE GILDED ROSEMARY LOLLIPOPS

Rosemary has been used at weddings since ancient times, to symbolise virility (Roman), faithfulness (Elizabethan), and as gilded sprigs to remind guests not to forget their loved ones (17th-century). Gilded rosemary lollipops are a lovely way to continue the tradition.

Makes 6–8 lollipops
200g (1 cup) granulated sugar
175ml (½ cup) raw runny honey
Handful of tender rosemary sprigs
Pinch of edible gold leaf flakes
Silicone 2.5cm (1in) heart or round-shaped multiple-cavity lollipop mould, plus wooden sticks

1 Place the sugar, honey and 4 tbsp of water in a medium pan. Bring to a boil. Stir until the sugar dissolves and the temperature reaches 150°C (300°F). Spoon a little mixture into cold water – it should produce hard candy strings.

2 Add tiny pieces of rosemary sprigs to the candy mix and quickly fill each lollipop mould. If necessary, use a toothpick to evenly arrange the herbs.

3 Press lollipop sticks in place and gently twist to coat entire surface with syrup. Leave to cool for at least 30 minutes.

4 Remove the lollipops from the moulds when the syrup is hard. Roll in a smattering of edible gold leaf.

5 Present the lollipops in a glass jar or pretty pot, or loosely wrap in baking parchment.

Other uses
❧ Place uplifting rosemary under your pillow to help promote calm, reduce anxiety or ward off bad dreams.
❧ Add a sprig of rosemary to a gin and tonic or the lime hit of a gimlet.

SORREL
Rumex, Polygonaceae family

Although 'There be divers kinds of Sorrel' (John Gerard, *Herball*, 1597) including the edible and medicinal common or garden sorrel (*Rumex acetosa*), smaller-leaved French or buckler leaf sorrel (*R. scutatus*) and wilder sheep's sorrel (*R. acetosella*), what they all have in common is a tart, sour green-apple taste due to high levels of oxalic acid. This compound – flavoursome and beneficial in small doses but toxic in larger amounts – also gives rhubarb and the non-related yet often juxtaposed wood sorrel (*Oxalis acetosella*) their pronounced flavour.

❧ THE DESCRIPTION Common or garden sorrel has deep roots, juicy red stems and lance-shaped leaves that often turn crimson towards the top. French sorrel is much prettier with squatter shield-shaped leaves, while sheep's sorrel has leaves shaped like barbed spears. All three are dioecious (male and female flowers on different plants), with blooms appearing as greenish spires, turning reddish brown as the fruit ripens.

❧ THE NAME The common name 'sorrel' stems from the Old French word *surrelle*, *sorele* or *sur* meaning 'sour', and the genus name *Rumex* from the Latin word *rumo* meaning 'to suck', in reference to the ancient practice of sucking on sorrel leaves to quench thirst. Pliny also refers to sorrel as *Lapatham* from the ancient Greek name *Lapathon*. *Acetosa* means 'acidic' and *scutatus* alludes to French sorrel's shield-like leaves.

❧ THE PLACE Common sorrel's native range extends across Europe, Eurasia and Asia but it has also naturalised in large pockets of North and South America, and Africa. Prolific sheep's sorrel now populates huge swathes of Europe, North America and South America, while French sorrel's native habitat is Central and southern Europe and temperate Asia. Plant sorrel in fertile soil in a bright spot out of the midday sun and grow French sorrel in large containers.

❧ THE TIME Sorrel blooms in mid-to-late summer, bringing warm blushes of reddish colour to the grassy spots where it grows wild. It is a cool-season perennial but is often grown as an annual. Divide mature plants in autumn or sow seed outside in late spring. Pick leaves when they are young and tender, removing flowers before they mature to keep a steady supply of edible foliage.

❧ THE VIRTUES Tudor-favourite common sorrel and French sorrel, introduced later, are both traditional salad herbs and used to flavour soups and ragoûts. Useful for 'all hot diseases', to 'cool any inflammation' and 'to quench thirst, and procure an appetite' (Nicholas Culpeper, *Complete Herbal*, 1653), sorrels are now known to be rich in vitamins C and A, plus iron, magnesium, potassium and calcium.

Plate 230.

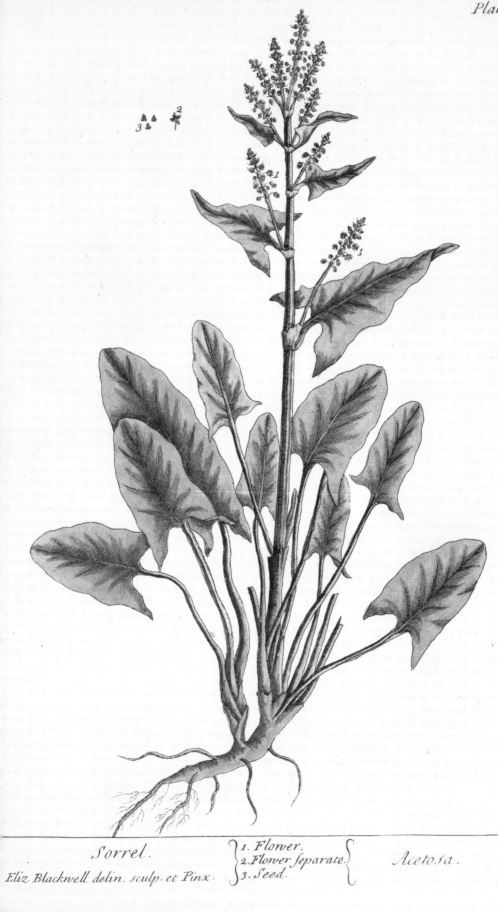

Sorrel.

1. Flower.
2. Flower separate.
3. Seed.

Acetosa.

Eliz. Blackwell delin. sculp. et Pinx.

HEAL
SORREL SOUP

Sour-tasting sorrel soup, known in Eastern European cuisines as *schav*, green *borscht* or green *shchi*, is packed with fibre, vitamins and minerals to help boost digestion and circulation.

Serves 6
Large bunch of common or French sorrel
1 onion
4 large potatoes
2 tbsp butter
1.5 litres (1½ quarts) vegetable stock
1 egg yolk
500ml (2 cups) *smetana* (thick sour cream) or crème fraîche, plus 6 tbsp to serve
Salt and pepper to taste
6 hard-boiled eggs, to serve

1 Wash and chop the sorrel. Finely dice the onion. Peel and cube the potatoes.

2 Cook the onion in the butter in a large pan until soft and golden. Stir in the potatoes, add the sorrel and cover with stock.

3 Simmer on a low heat for around 15 minutes, or until the potato is tender. Remove from the heat and leave to cool a little. Purée with a stick blender.

4 Whisk the egg yolk and *smetana* or créme fraîche in a bowl. Whisk in one quarter of the soup to temper, then transfer the mixture to the main pan. Keep whisking on a low heat for around 5 minutes until the soup thickens.

5 Serve hot, with a dollop of *smetana* or crème fraiche and a halved boiled egg in each bowl.

Other uses
♣ Place a sorrel leaf over a mouth ulcer to help soothe pain and stimulate healing.
♣ Sip on a vitamin- and mineral-rich infusion of fresh or dried sorrel leaves or use cooled as a facial toner or hair rinse.

NOURISH
SORREL SAUCE

Use bright, lemony sorrel to add an extra punch to soups, sauces or plainer dishes. A classic pairing is shredded common or French sorrel with cream or crème fraîche in a hot buttery sauce. Perfect drizzled over poached eggs, in an omelette, with pasta or with grilled vegetables.

Serves 2
Large bunch of fresh common or French sorrel
1 tbsp butter
1 heaped tbsp crème fraîche or double cream
1 egg yolk (optional)
Salt and pepper to taste

1 Wash the sorrel and remove any tough stalks. Shred the leaves by rolling into cigar shapes and slicing thinly.

2 Melt the butter in a pan, stir in the shredded sorrel and wilt for a few seconds. Aim to keep something of the bright green colour.

3 Stir in the crème fraîche or double cream. Cook for around 1 minute. Add salt and pepper to taste.

4 For a richer flavour and consistency, beat in an egg yolk, turn off the heat and seal with a lid. Keep warm until ready to serve.

Other uses
♣ Blend 100g (4 cups) of sorrel, 125g (½ cup) of yogurt, a garlic clove, 1 tbsp of olive oil and 1 tsp of Dijon mustard to make a tangy dressing, dip or drizzle.
♣ Create a piquant summer salad or flatbread sandwich of fresh sorrel, hot peppery watercress, goat's cheese and thin slices of fresh orange.

STYLE
SORREL SMOOTHIE

Start the day with an uplifting, nutritious blend of fresh, zesty sorrel leaves, smooth avocado, banana and almond or oat milk. Bring out sorrel's natural citrus flavour with an extra squeeze of lemon, or try adding fruit such as strawberries or kiwi fruit. The smoothie can also be served over ice as a refreshing summer drink.

Makes 1 smoothie
Handful of fresh common or French sorrel
1 banana
½ avocado
250ml (1 cup) almond or oat milk
1 lemon

1 Wash and shred the sorrel. Chop the banana and avocado. Add to a blender.

2 Add the almond or oat milk.

3 Blend well to create a lovely green liquid. Add a squeeze of lemon to taste.

Other uses
❧ Add ornamental interest to the herb patch by growing red-veined sorrel (*Rumex sanguineus*) as well as common and French sorrel. All are good harvested as micro-herbs for garnishing.
❧ Make a science meets art, Emily Dickinson-style herbarium of locally grown and gathered plants, mounting contrasting species of *Rumex* side to side – press extra samples to mount as botanical art.

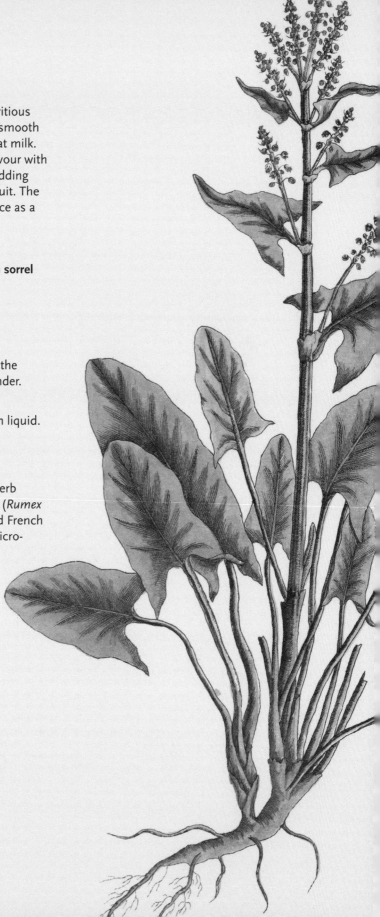

SAGE
Salvia officinalis, Lamiaceae family

Common or garden sage (*Salvia officinalis*) has been hailed for its medicinal and culinary properties since ancient times. The familiar bushy shrub with soft, grey-green hairy leaves, blue-purple flowers and a warm, minty-floral aroma and taste now has numerous forms with foliage and flowers in various shades, helping to establish sage as an attractive garden plant. Although thankfully no longer used to ward off the Plague, it is still a traditional herbal remedy for sore throats, wind, depression and fever, as well as a strong, earthy culinary seasoning.

❀ **THE DESCRIPTION** Spreading, evergreen sage has woody stems, finely veined, paired aromatic leaves and two-lipped flowers in spiked whorls. Popular forms include 'Purpurascens' (purple foliage), 'Tricolor' (variegated green, pink and white) and 'Aurea' (yellow leaved), while close relatives include similarly medicinal and culinary *Salvia fruticosa* (Greek sage) and therapeutic *S. sclarea* (clary sage).

❀ **THE NAME** *Salvia* stems from the Latin word *salvere* meaning 'to be saved', pointing to sage's historical use as a cure-all. This was then corrupted to the Old French *Sauge* and Old English *Sawge* leading to the common name sage. Previous synonyms include the Ancient Greek *Sphakos* or *Elelisphakos*, thought to be wild and cultivated sage respectively, plus *Salvia salvatrix* meaning 'sage the saviour'.

❀ **THE PLACE** Both common sage (*Salvia officinalis*) and Greek sage (*S. fruticosa*) are native to the Mediterranean region, including parts of Greece, Italy and Spain. A long history of introduction and cultivation, however, has since extended their reach to North America, the Middle East and North Africa, plus gardens around the world. Grow sage in light, well-drained soil in a sunny yet sheltered spot that is not too wet in winter.

❀ **THE TIME** Sage is best propagated by softwood cuttings in spring, semi-ripe cuttings in late summer, or by layering (pegging a long sage stem to the soil to encourage new roots to form). It flowers in midsummer and can be harvested all year round, clipping just above the spot where two leaves meet. For the most aromatic leaves, harvest in the morning once the dew has dried.

❀ **THE VIRTUES** Mrs M. Grieve includes several varieties of sage in *A Modern Herbal* (1931) plus numerous folk remedies and recipes including sage tea, sage vinegar, sage tooth powder, sage and onion sauce, a sore throat gargle and a cure for sprains. Sage is now known to be rich in antioxidants and to have antimicrobial properties, as well as making the best-tasting stuffing.

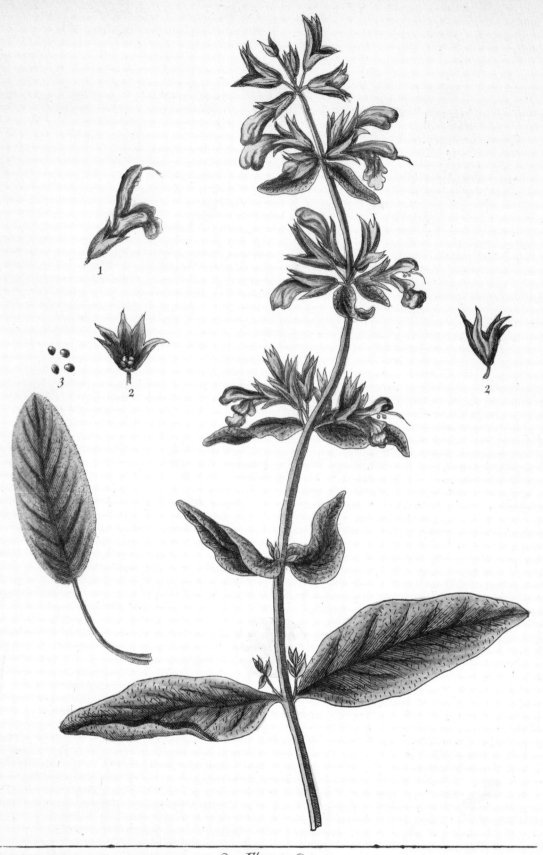

Sage

1 Flower
2 Fruit
3 Seed

Salvia

HEAL SAGE HOT-FLUSH TINCTURE

Sage extract or tincture has been used for centuries as a folk remedy for reducing fever and perspiration. It is thought to lessen the effects of menopause-related hot flushes and night sweats.

Fills up to 5 x 100ml (3½fl oz) dropper bottles
1 large bunch of fresh sage
500ml (2 cups) 80–90 per cent proof vodka

1 Remove the sage leaves from the stalks. Discard the stalks. Wash the leaves and lay out on a cloth to dry overnight.

2 Chop the leaves and place in a sterilized 500ml (17½fl oz) glass lidded jar. Cover the herbs entirely with the vodka almost to the top.

3 Seal with a lid and leave in a cool, dark place for 4–6 weeks. Shake the jar every 2–3 days. Ensure the herbs stay covered.

4 Strain the tincture through muslin into a glass bowl. Cover and leave to stand overnight. Strain again.

5 Use a funnel to decant the tincture into sterilised 100ml (3½fl oz) amber-coloured glass dropper bottles. Label and store in a dark place.

6 Adult doses are 30–60 drops (1–5ml or 1/5–1 tsp) tincture in a little water, twice a day.

Other uses
❧ Sip on a sage leaf infusion – helpful to stimulate and boost the appetite when recovering from illness or feeling weak. Avoid if breastfeeding.
❧ Sage oxymel, made from sage leaves, honey and apple cider vinegar, can be soothing for sore throats, coughs, fevers or indigestion.

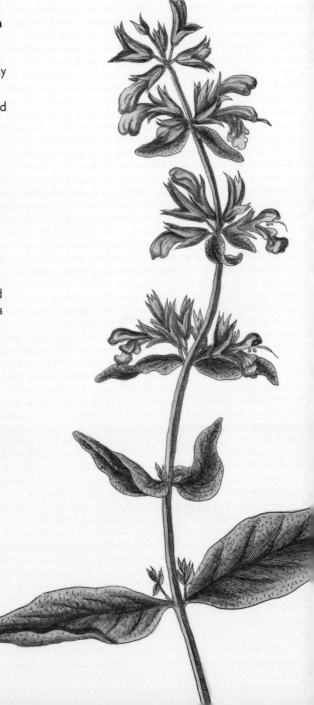

NOURISH SAGE AND ONION STUFFING

Grains, breadcrumbs, herbs and onions have been combined to cook within meat, fish or vegetables since humans first learned to roast over a fire. Sage and onion stuffing is a particularly well-known classic, traditionally served up at Christmas, Thanksgiving or as part of a weekly Sunday roast.

Serves 6
1 white onion
Large handful of fresh sage leaves
1 egg
75g (2½oz) butter
90g (3oz) fresh white breadcrumbs
Sea salt and black pepper to taste

1 Pre-heat the oven to 190°C (375°F). Finely dice the onion. Finely chop the sage leaves. Beat the egg in bowl.

2 Heat the butter in a pan and gently sweat the onion until translucent.

3 Transfer the onion to a bowl and add the sage and breadcrumbs, then sea salt and black pepper to taste.

4 Mix in the beaten egg. Use your hands to roll the mixture into small stuffing balls.

5 Place the balls on a non-stick baking tray and cook for 30 minutes. Use to stuff a roast or serve as a herby side dish.

Other uses
❧ Fry fresh sage leaves in a little hot olive oil for 2–3 seconds or until crisp. Pat dry, sprinkle with sea salt and serve with pasta or as a garnish for soup.
❧ Make a sage leaf and virgin olive oil infusion to provide an aromatic dip for bread or a drizzle for roasts or bakes.

STYLE PURIFYING SMOKE STICK

Herbs have been burned to help cleanse or purify the home for millennia, the most well-known being sacred white sage (*Salvia apiana*) used in Native American smudging ceremonies. Burn bundles of garden sage, rosemary and lavender to help freshen a room, repel insects and channel positive, plant-inspired energy.

Makes 1 purifying stick
Small bunch of dried sage
Small bunch of dried lavender
Small bunch of dried rosemary
Small handful of dried rose petals
1m (3ft) natural jute twine

1 Harvest the sage, lavender and rosemary stems. Dry in loose bunches upside down (see pages 16–17). Harvest the rose buds. Dry the petals on a tray.

2 Bundle the herbs together, sandwiching rose petals between longer plant parts. Wind twine around the bundle to secure, starting at the base and keeping a few pretty rose petals on the outside.

3 Criss-cross the twine back down to the base and finish with a knot.

4 Light the tip of the herb bundle, wafting aromatic smoke around the room to cleanse and balance.

Other uses
❧ Garnish drinks or canapés with other attractive sages, including tangy pineapple sage (*Salvia elegans*), red-flowered, sweet blackcurrant sage (*S. microphylla*) or variegated sage (*S. officinalis* 'Tricolor').
❧ Combine fresh sage leaves with equal parts white vinegar and distilled water to make an antibacterial, antimicrobial home-cleaning spray.

ELDER

Sambucus nigra, Adoxaceae family

'It has been said, with some truth, that our English summer is not here until the Elder is fully in flower, and that it ends when the berries are ripe', writes Mrs M. Grieve in *A Modern Herbal* (1931) of this lacy-flowered, jewel-berried scrubland stalwart. Once regarded as a rural 'medicine chest', various parts of the common elder (*Sambucus nigra*) have been used for centuries to remedy ailments from colds and fever to 'dropsy' (oedema) and grey hair. Recipes also abound for tasty and potentially immune-boosting robs (see overleaf), syrups, cordials, wines, jams, jellies and ketchups, plus perfumed elderflower cordials and cocktails.

❧ **THE DESCRIPTION** The appearance of this hardy hedgerow shrub with furrowed bark and large, serrated leaves that give off a 'ranke and stinking smell' (John Gerard, *Herball*, 1597) is somewhat unremarkable. Its appearance is transformed, however, when the flat-topped, creamy-white, fragrant blossoms appear, followed by drooping bunches of shiny purplish-black berries.

❧ **THE NAME** Shrouded in folklore, romance and superstition, the common name 'elder' stems from the Anglo-Saxon word *aeld* meaning fire, harking back to the ancient practice of using hollowed out stems to blow on flames. The generic name *Sambucus* can be traced back to Roman times, one theory linking it to an ancient musical instrument, while the species *nigra* relates to the black tone of the berries.

❧ **THE PLACE** Native to western and eastern Europe and parts of Eurasia, *Sambucus nigra* is now found in northern Europe, North Africa, western Asia and parts of South America, flourishing in both urban and countryside habitats. To cultivate, grow in moderately fertile, humus-rich, moist but well-drained soil in full sun or dappled shade; elder also fares well on an extremely chalky site.

❧ **THE TIME** Elderflowers, according to Mrs M. Grieve, should be collected in midsummer 'when just in full bloom'. Left in a warm place 'the corollas become loosened and can then be removed by sifting'; the creamy fragrance also develops at this time. Harvest elderberries in late summer through early autumn to use fresh or dried. Propagate by softwood cuttings in early summer or hardwood cuttings in winter.

❧ **THE VIRTUES** The leaves, stems, sap and bark of the common elder were traditionally employed to purge a fever or expel phlegm or 'choler' (angry bile). Purging was probably the effect of a toxic cyanide-inducing glycoside now known to exist in high quantities in elder's leaves and stalks. Focus instead on the antioxidant immune-boosting berries and sweet, delicately-scented flowers.

Plate 151.

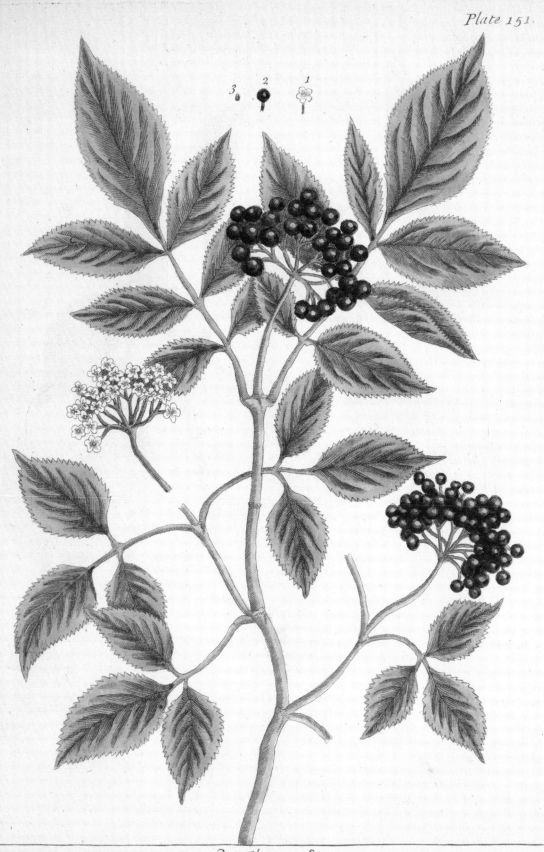

3   2   1

Elder.   } 1. Flower. {
                             } 2. Berry. {   *Sambucus.*
Eliz. Blackwell delin. sculp. et Pinx. } 3. Seed. {

HEAL
ELDERBERRY ROB SYRUP

Combine a traditional elder rob (from the Arabic *robb* meaning boiled down juice of a fruit or vegetable) with an elder syrup (from the Arabic *sharáb*, essentially a sweetened-up rob) to help remedy a cough or congestion.

Makes 2 x 250ml (8fl oz) bottles
450g (1lb) fresh ripe elderberries (with stalks removed), or 225g (8oz) dried elderberries
250g (9oz) granulated sugar or 175g (6oz) raw runny honey
5 whole cloves
2.5cm (1in) cube fresh ginger, grated
1 cinnamon stick
2 tsp dried lemon or orange peel

1 If using fresh elderberries, wash thoroughly to remove insects. Pat dry and, if possible, freeze for several hours before stripping berries from stalks using a fork. Remove all traces of stalk. Leave to defrost.

2 Place the fresh or dried berries in a pan. Smash fresh berries with a fork to release juice. Cover with cold water.

3 Bring to a boil, then simmer for around 35–40 minutes until reduced to around 500ml (17½fl oz) of elder rob (condensed juice). Strain through a muslin cloth into a jug, then return the liquid to the pan. Compost berry remnants.

4 Add the sugar or honey, the cinnamon stick, ginger and citrus peel. Simmer until syrupy. Leave to cool slightly

5 Decant into hot 250ml (8fl oz) sterilised airtight glass bottles leaving a 1cm (½in) gap at the top. Seal with a bung. Store in the fridge unopened for 3 months, opened for 3–4 weeks. Take 10ml (2 tsp) of immune-boosting syrup three times a day or add 15ml (1 tbsp) to 250ml (1 cup) of just-boiled water for a warming drink.

Other uses
❧ Make vitamin C-rich tea by simmering 2 tbsp of dried elderberries in 250ml (1 cup) of water for 20 minutes.
❧ Prepare a potent elderberry tincture by steeping fresh elderberries in vodka in an airtight jar for 6 weeks.

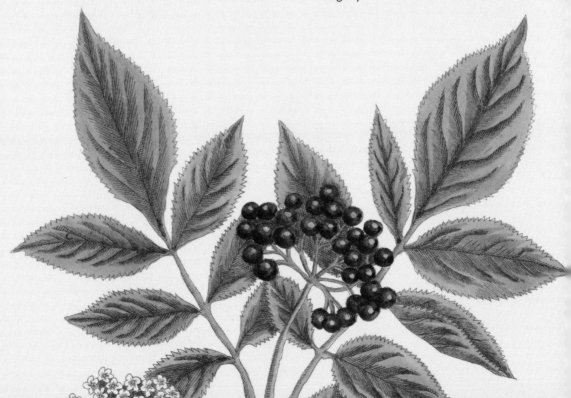

NOURISH
ELDERBERRY JELLY

Slightly tweaked, elderberry rob syrup becomes a health-giving and delicious jelly. Eat on toast or croissants, in porridge or yogurt, use as a glaze for roasts, in cakes or other baked goods, in salad dressings or sauces, or as the pièce de résistance of a cheeseboard.

Makes approx. 2 x 300ml (10½fl oz) jars jelly
500ml (2 cups) elder rob (see recipe and method opposite)
2 tbsp pure pectin
200g (1 cup) white granulated sugar
Juice of 1 lemon

1 Follow steps 1–3 for the Elderberry Rob Syrup, but let the juice strain slowly through a jelly bag into a large non-reactive pan overnight.

2 Add the pectin to the juice and whisk until dissolved. Then add the sugar and lemon juice and bring to a boil. Simmer for around 4 minutes, or according to the instructions on the pectin box.

3 Remove the jelly from the heat and allow it to stand for around 5 minutes.

4 Decant into two 300ml (10½fl oz) sterilised airtight jars. Store in a cool, dark place unopened for 2 years; opened in the fridge for 2–3 months. Use as a spread, in porridge, or in cooking or baking as desired.

Other uses
❧ Combine elderberries, blackberries, haws and crab apples with sugar, salt, vinegar, shallots and spices to make a savoury hedgerow ketchup.
❧ Make a traditional elderberry pie offsetting the tangy berry filling with a buttery pastry lattice top.

STYLE
ELDERFLOWER CORDIAL

This traditional summer drink can be traced back to Roman times and is perfect for al fresco gatherings or weddings. Harvest elderflowers on a warm morning in midsummer from a non-polluted spot and selecting blossoms that have just opened. Keep flowers upright to preserve the fragrant pollen and store in a warm place to help bring out the perfume.

Makes 2 x 500ml (17½fl oz) bottles
15 elderflower heads
2 lemons (unwaxed)
1kg (5 cups) caster sugar
30g (1oz) citric acid

1 Wash the elderflowers thoroughly and remove as much of the green stem as possible. Zest the lemons, then peel and finely slice the fruit.

2 Place the sugar and 1 litre (1 quart) of water in a large pan and bring to a boil, stirring until the sugar is dissolved. Add the lemon zest and citric acid and stir again. Remove from the heat.

3 Place the elderflowers in a bowl, add the lemon slices and submerge with the syrup. Cover with a cloth and leave for 24 hours.

4 Strain the liquid through muslin into a large jug. Then funnel into two sterilised airtight 500ml (17½fl oz) bottles. Store in a cool dark place for 2 months, opened in the fridge for 4 weeks, or freeze in ice-cube trays. Dilute with sparkling or still water or use in cocktails or desserts.

Other uses
❧ Fry washed elderflowers (stalks removed) in a light tempura batter served with blossom honey or sugar and cinnamon – an ideal party canapé.
❧ Make a beautiful blue cyanotype artwork by laying lacy elderflower blooms and leaves over sun-sensitive paper.

SALAD BURNET

Sanguisorba minor, Rosaceae family

Serrated-leaved, blood-red flowered salad burnet (*Sanguisorba minor*) is the best-known species of *Sanguisorba*. Its cucumber-flavoured leaves have been used as an edible kitchen garden herb and salad, as well as medicinally, for hundreds of years. Often mentioned in herbals alongside great burnet (*S officinalis*) – another stalwart of the traditional first-aid kit for its similar potential to stem wounds – these two are now often used alongside other tall flowering, ornamental *Sanguisorba* genera in naturalistic garden plantings.

❀ THE DESCRIPTION Salad burnet's freshly scented, clump-forming leaflets are 'more numerous, five to ten pairs, and shorter than those of the Great Burnet. The flowers in each head bear crimson tufted stigmas, the lower ones thirty to forty stamens, with very long, dropping filaments. Both the flower and leafstalks are a deep-crimson colour' (Mrs M. Grieve, *A Modern Herbal*, 1931). Great burnet is taller, with deep purple-brown flowers.

❀ THE NAME Dioscorides (*De Materia Medica*, AD 50–70) records a type of edible, medicinal herb thought to be salad or great burnet as *Poterion*, alluding to its historic preparation in a 'goblet' of wine. The burnets were later assigned to the genus *Pimpinella*, great burnet's former species name. The current genus name *Sanguisorba* means 'to absorb blood', a reference to its past use on the battlefield.

❀ THE PLACE *Sanguisorba minor* is native to the grassy meadows of Europe, northern Africa and temperate Asia, and has naturalised in northern Eurasia, Australia and the Americas. *S. officinalis* is native to a huge range of the northern temperate hemisphere including North America and China where it is known as the herb *Di Yu*. Both will grow in moderately fertile, well-drained soil in full sun or partial shade.

❀ THE TIME Salad burnet is a herbaceous perennial that can be propagated by seed or by division in autumn. The leaves remain green throughout much of the year, providing an ample harvest but may taste bitter in hot summers. *Sanguisorba* flowers bloom well above the foliage from early summer through autumn, followed by burred fruit.

❀ THE VIRTUES On the ancient battlefields of Greece and Rome, burnet's naturally astringent roots or leaves were used to staunch wounds. Considered the ideal health-boosting garnish for wine or eaten as a nutritious salad leaf – it is now known to be packed with antioxidants and vitamin C – burnet is one herb that should always have its place, as it did 'In the herb gardens of older days' (*A Modern Herbal*, 1931).

Plate 413.

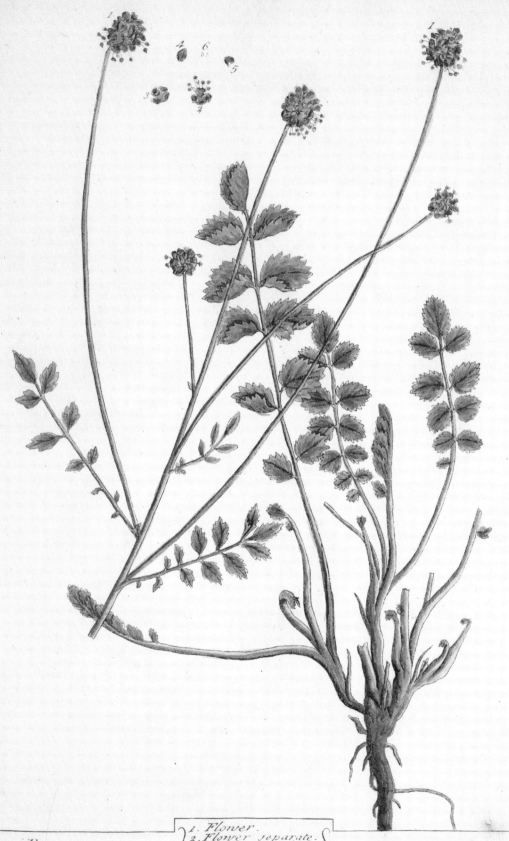

Burnet.   Pimpinella.

1. Flower.
2. Flower separate.
3. Back of the Flower.
4. Seed Vessel.
5. Seed Vessel open.
6. Seed.

Eliz. Blackwell delin. sculp. et Pinx.

HEAL
FIRST-AID POULTICE

Naturally astringent, cooling salad burnet has the potential to act as a styptic – a substance that can help stop bleeding, as its genus name *Sanguisorba* suggests. Verdant, easily pounded and in leaf for most of the year, it's an ideal go-to for treating minor cuts and bruises.

Makes 1 poultice
Large handful of salad burnet leaves
1 tbsp distilled water
Cotton bandage

1 Use a pestle and mortar to grind the leaves. Add the water to help release the juices.

2 Clean the minor cut with water and place the macerated leaves onto the affected area. Hold in place with a bandage and leave for a few hours to let the herbal benefits penetrate the skin.

3 Remove the poultice and gently wash and dry the skin.

Other uses
♣ Steep a small handful of torn salad burnet leaves in 250ml (1 cup) of just-boiled water. Sip as a digestion-boosting, vitamin-C-rich aperitif.
♣ Decant a cooled infusion of salad burnet into a spray bottle to use as a refreshing, astringent facial spray for hot days or while travelling.

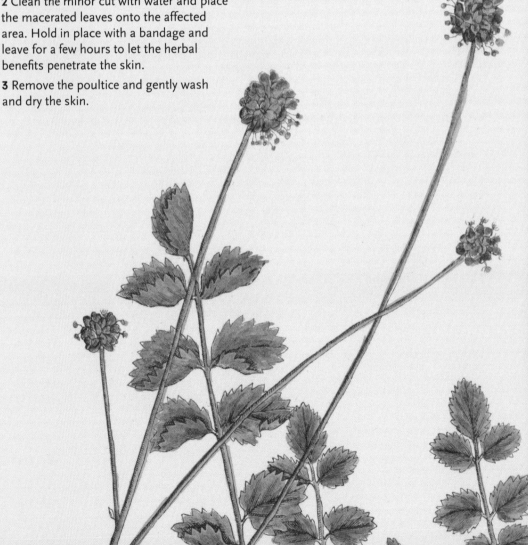

NOURISH SALAD BURNET VINEGAR AND VINAIGRETTE

Salad burnet, a favourite Elizabethan and Victorian herb, adds a fresh, floral, slight cucumber note to vinegar. Delicious as the base for a zesty vinaigrette dressing.

Makes 1 x 500ml (17½fl oz) bottle
For the salad burnet vinegar:
Large bunch of stalked salad burnet leaves, plus extra (chopped) for the vinaigrette
500ml (2 cups) white wine vinegar

For the vinaigrette:
3 tbsp salad burnet vinegar (see above)
125ml (½ cup) olive oil
Zest of 1 lemon
Sea salt and black pepper

1 To make the vinegar, pack the salad burnet leaves and stalks into a sterilised 1 litre (1 quart) lidded glass jar until half full. Push down with a pestle to bruise the leaves slightly.

2 Cover the burnet with the white wine vinegar. Close with a lid.

3 Leave to macerate for a week in a warm place. Strain through muslin into a sterilised 500ml (17½fl oz) glass bottle.

4 Seal with a bung or add a pouring nozzle for easy drizzling. Store in a fridge for up to 6 months.

5 To make the vinaigrette dressing, combine the infused vinegar with the olive oil. Add the lemon zest and salt and pepper to taste. Add a few more salad burnet leaves for extra zing.

Other use
♣ Fold fresh salad burnet leaves into cream cheese as a refreshing filling for sandwiches or baked potatoes.

STYLE GARDEN GIMLET

Salad burnet was traditionally floated on wine to help stave off illness and promote joy. Extend the tradition by adding salad burnet syrup to summer cocktails, such as this zingy, slightly bitter Garden Gimlet.

Makes 2 cocktails
For the salad burnet syrup:
200g (1 cup) granulated sugar
Small bunch of salad burnet (leaves and stems)

For the Garden Gimlet:
4 sprigs of salad burnet
1 tbsp salad burnet syrup (see above)
Juice of 2 limes
120ml (4fl oz) dry gin
3 cracked ice cubes

1 Place 250ml (1 cup) of water and the sugar in a pan. Bring to a boil then simmer until dissolved.

2 Allow the syrup to cool a little. Add the salad burnet, setting a couple of sprigs aside to garnish. Cover and steep for 30 minutes. Strain through muslin into a sterilised 250ml (8fl oz) lidded glass jar.

3 For the Gimlet, muddle three of the four sprigs of salad burnet and the salad burnet syrup in a cocktail shaker.

4 Add the lime juice, gin and 3 cracked ice cubes and shake.

5 Strain into two 200ml (7fl oz) martini glasses. Garnish with a salad burnet sprigs.

Other uses
♣ Create a knot garden using red-flowered salad burnet as a filler among hedges of rosemary or lavender.
♣ Encase sprigs of salad burnet leaves within ice cubes for a vibrant green addition to drinks.

SAVORY
Satureja, Lamiaceae family

Within the *Satureja* species, the most familiar are the peppery-tasting, perennial winter savory (*Satureja montana*) and the bushier, more delicately flavoured annual summer savory (*S. hortensis*). Both have a long history of culinary and medicinal use to help prevent or calm wind – they are often found in dishes containing beans – treat insect bites or stings (a remedy still reputed to be used by gardeners today), as a highly aromatic stewing or flavouring herb, and even as an aphrodisiac. All excellent reasons to add winter or summer savory to your herb patch.

❧ THE DESCRIPTION Winter savory is a dwarf, shrubby perennial with lance-shaped, dark green aromatic leaves and dense spikes of small, whorled, two-lipped light-purple to white or pink flowers. Annual summer savory has bronze-green leaves and white to mauve blooms. Other notable species are Greek, pink-flowered savory (*Satureja thymbra*) and white-flowered creeping savory (*S. spicigera*).

❧ THE NAME The etymology of the genus name *Satureja* (previously *Satureia*) is unclear, although links to ancient Greek *satyrs* – lustful woodland gods said to use summer savory as an aphrodisiac – and the herb mix *za'atar* (see page 105) abound. *Montana* and *hortensis* mean 'of the mountains' and 'of the garden' respectively, although both species of savory have been cultivated in gardens for centuries.

❧ THE PLACE Summer savory's native range extends from southeast Europe to southwest Siberia, although it has been introduced to other parts of Europe and parts of North America. Winter savory is native to temperate regions of southern Europe, the Mediterranean and Africa but has also been much more widely introduced. Grow either species in light, well-drained soil in beds or containers in full sun.

❧ THE TIME Propagate perennial winter savory by softwood cuttings in summer. Harvest leaves year-round, ideally on a summer morning when dew has dried. Sow annual summer savory under cover in early spring and transplant after the last frost. Harvest in summer when it is at least 15cm (6in) tall; snip leaves and shoots from mature stalks. Plant summer savory with broad beans to boost growth by repelling pests.

❧ THE VIRTUES Elizabeth Blackwell (*A Curious Herbal*, 1737–39) lists both winter and summer savory as 'esteem'd heating, drying and carminative, good to expel Wind from the Stomach and Bowels, ease the Asthma and Affections of the Breast, open Obstructions of the Womb, and promote the Menses'. Both savories are now known to be highly antioxidant and potentially antibacterial and antifungal due to the presence of thymol and carvacrol.

Plate 318.

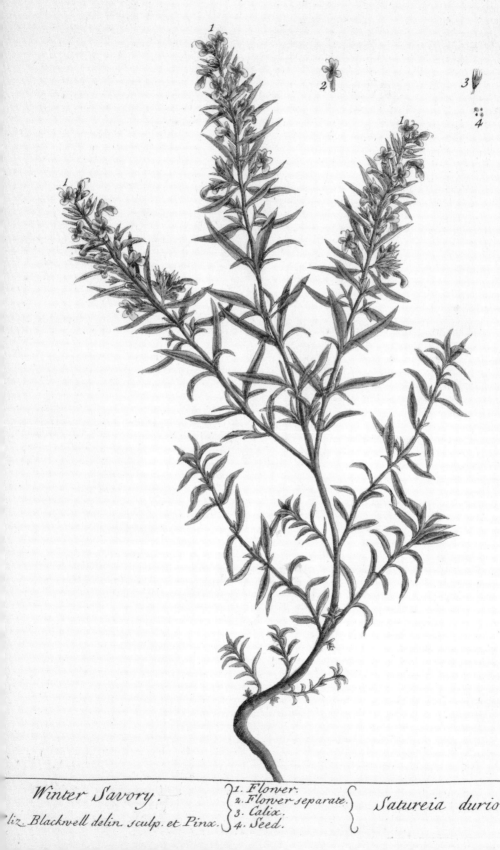

Winter Savory.

1. *Flower.*
2. *Flower separate.*
3. *Calix.*
4. *Seed.*

Satureia durior.

liz. Blackwell delin. sculp. et Pinx.

HEAL
NATURAL BITE RELIEF

Naturally antiseptic, anti-inflammatory savory has been used for centuries as a natural first aid treatment for insect bites and stings. A sprig was placed directly onto the sore area or the leaves crushed into a soothing poultice. Include a bush of winter or summer savory in your garden so that you always have some to hand.

Makes 1 poultice
Large handful of fresh winter or summer savory sprigs
Cotton bandage

1 Strip the leaves from the stalks and use a pestle and mortar to grind down. Add up to 1 tbsp of the water to help get the juices flowing.

2 Place the poultice on the bite or sting. Hold in place with a bandage until soothed.

3 Remove the poultice and gently wash and dry the skin.

Other uses
❧ Make a digestive and appetite-stimulating tea by infusing 250ml (1 cup) just-boiled water with 4 tbsp of dried summer or winter savory.
❧ Add a few drops of naturally expectorant winter savory essential oil to steaming hot water to use as a decongestant inhalation.

NOURISH
HERBES DE PROVENCE

Herbes de Provence, a mix popularised in the 1970s, takes its inspiration from herbs growing in the Provence region of southeast France. The exact combination is not defined but typically includes savory, marjoram, thyme and oregano, plus tarragon and fennel. Culinary lavender is often added for an extra layer of Provençal flavour and charm.

Makes 1 x 125ml (4½fl oz) jar
1 tbsp fennel seeds (optional)
2 tbsp fresh rosemary leaves
4 tbsp dried thyme leaves
3 tbsp dried marjoram leaves
3 tbsp dried summer savory leaves
1 tbsp dried oregano leaves
1 tbsp dried tarragon leaves (optional)
1 tsp lavender buds (optional)

1 Grind and crush the fennel seeds and rosemary using a pestle and mortar. Pour into a small mixing bowl.

2 Add the remaining herbs. Mix well and transfer to an airtight 125ml (4½oz) glass lidded jar.

Other uses
❧ The Romans used winter savory to impart a salt-and-pepper flavour to their food – ideal for those trying to remove sodium from their diet.
❧ Naturally carminative summer savory, known as *Bohnenkraut* ('bean herb') in German, is a great addition to bean stews or soups.

STYLE
SAVORY LOVE POTION

Savory has been a popular ingredient in love potions from ancient Rome up to the 20th century when French herbalist Maurice Méssegué perpetuated the belief that summer savory was a love-boosting 'herb of happiness'. Keep the myth alive.

Makes 1 x 50ml (1¾fl oz) potion
Large bunch of fresh summer savory
50ml (1¾fl oz) bottle with cork or cap
Small natural card tag on twine

1 Harvest summer savory on a dry morning. Hang in a loose bunch, upside down to dry.

2 Strip dried savory leaves from the stalks. Reduce to a fine powder using a herb grinder or pestle and mortar.

3 Place the powder in the glass bottle and seal.

4 Label the 'Savory Love Potion' by attaching the tag and perhaps add a little handwritten scroll detailing its aphrodisiac uses, such as sprinkling on meals or a Bloody Mary.

5 Make a batch of the potion to offer wedding guests, or present a jar to your chosen one as a gesture of love.

Other uses
❧ Macerate a handful of fresh summer savory in red wine vinegar for a week, then decant into a bottle as a flavoursome gift.
❧ Combine dried summer or winter savory with dried hops or lavender in a sleep-enhancing dreamtime pillow.

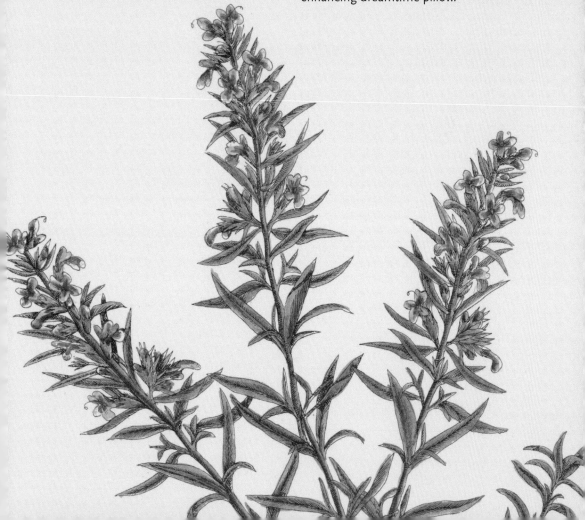

DANDELION
Taraxacum officinale, Asteraceae family

This yellow-flowered, tooth-leaved, tap-rooted, persistent ubiquitous and tenacious perennial receives high praises in the canon of herbals. Nicholas Culpeper alludes to flavoursome and nutritious qualities that make the 'French and Dutch so often eat them in the Spring' (*Complete Herbal*, 1653), while Mrs M. Grieve (*A Modern Herbal*, 1931) offers a range of recipes and remedies made with all parts of this abundant plant from 'excellent salads' and 'delicious sandwiches' to 'digestive drinks' and 'Dandelion Coffee'. Time, perhaps to welcome this troublesome weed back into the garden.

❦ THE DESCRIPTION John Parkinson (*Theatrum Botanicum*, 1640) describes common dandelion as 'well knowne to have many long and deeply gashed leaves lying on the ground round about the head of the roote' with 'stalkes, every one of them bearing at the toppe one large yellow flower' which 'becometh as round as a ball with long reddish seede ... blowne away with the wind'. The overall taste is bitter like rocket.

❦ THE NAME The word dandelion stems from the French *dent-de-lion* from the Latin *dens leonis* meaning 'lion's tooth' on account of the serrated leaves. While the genus word *Taraxacum* is thought to derive from the Arabic word *tarakhshaqun*, referring to a 'bitter herb'. Both *officinale* and the 'vulgarly called piss-a-beds' (*Complete Herbal*, 1653) refer to dandelion's use as a medicinal herb and its diuretic effect.

❦ THE PLACE Dandelions are thought to have evolved millions of years ago and were well known to the ancient Egyptians, Persians, Greeks, Romans and Chinese. Thanks to human introduction, they can now be found in nearly every country in the world including tropical, mountainous and arctic zones. Let flowers set seed and they will establish in almost any ground.

❦ THE TIME Dandelion leaves, roots and flowers are all edible. Harvest young leaves, before flowering, in early spring when they are less bitter; the blooms between spring and autumn each year; and the root between autumn and winter when the plant is dormant and the nutrients stored. The time from flowering to seed is roughly 9–12 days.

❦ THE VIRTUES First recorded in the ancient Chinese *Tang Materia Medica* (659 BC), the humble dandelion is now known to be rich in protein, potassium, calcium and vitamins A, C, E and B, and can be beneficial as a diuretic, detoxifier and skin tonic. The blooms also provide an ideal pollen and nectar pit-stop for bees, while the puffball clocks are inspiring for kids' play and botanical crafting.

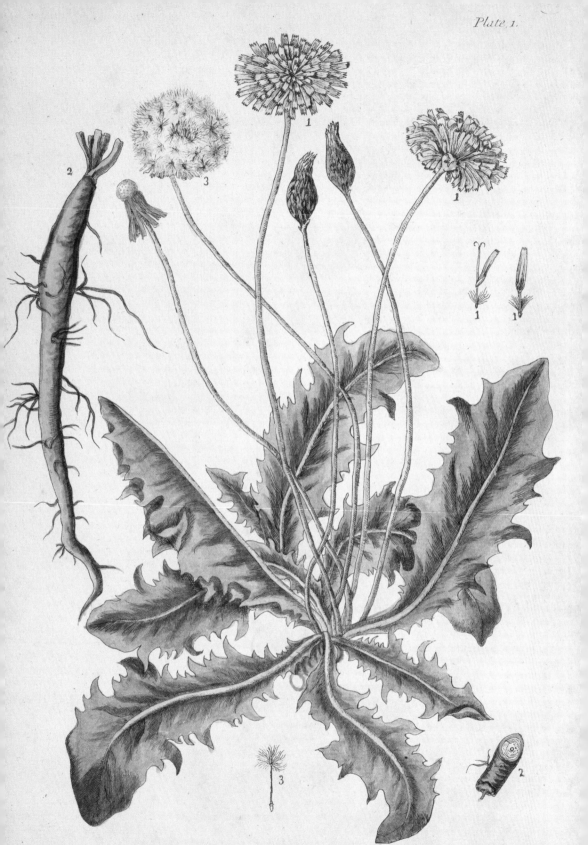

Dandelion

{ 1 Flower }
{ 2 Root }
{ 3 Seed }

Dens Leonis
Taraxacum

Eliz. Blackwell delin. sculp. et Pinx.

HEAL
DANDELION WINE

Imbibed as a delicious drink or taken as a daily detoxifying tonic, this warm, earthy wine is a wonderful way to celebrate dandelion's bold first flush of spring.

Makes around 4.5 litres (1 gallon)
Large tote bag of dandelion flowers
4.5 litres (1 gallon) just-boiled, distilled water
Zest and juice of 3 lemons
1 tbsp freshly grated ginger
1.5kg (6 cups) granulated sugar
450g (1lb) golden sultanas (crushed)
1 sachet wine yeast
1 tsp yeast nutrient

1 Wash the dandelion petals (minus the green bases) and place in a large non-reactive pan. Cover with the water and leave for 2 days.

2 Add the lemon zest and ginger. Bring to a boil. Stir in the sugar, remove from the heat and add the sultanas and lemon juice.

3 Pour the mixture into a sterile 10 litre (2 gallon) fermentation bucket. Add the wine yeast and yeast nutrient and cover with a tea towel. Ferment for 3–4 days. Stir daily.

4 Strain through three layers of muslin into a 5 litre (1 gallon) glass demi-john with an airlock (bubble trap) device. Allow to ferment for several months until no further bubbles are released.

5 Siphon into smaller 1 litre (1 quart) bottles and seal. Drink as wine or serve a shot a day as a health-boosting tonic.

Other uses
❧ Prepare a mineral-rich dandelion infusion with a little sugar to counteract bitterness.
❧ Soothe cracked skin with a dandelion-flower-infused salve.

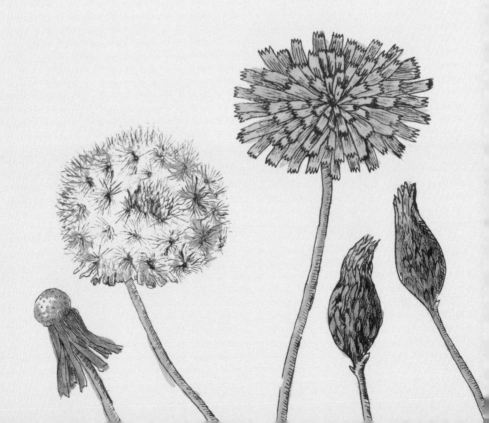

NOURISH
ZESTY DANDELION SALAD

The best and easiest way to eat dandelion greens is in an earthy, zesty salad combined with other early spring offerings such as wild garlic (*Allium ursinum*) or garlic scapes – the immature flower stalks of hardneck garlic (*Allium sativum*) plants.

Serves 2
Large bunch of tender dandelion leaves
1 tbsp finely chopped wild garlic or garlic scapes
1 tbsp lemon juice
½ tsp sea salt
¼ tsp granulated sugar
3½ tbsp extra virgin olive oil

1 Pick tender dandelion leaves from a non-polluted spot. Wash thoroughly. Arrange in a salad bowl.

2 Combine the wild garlic or garlic scapes with the lemon juice, salt and sugar in a bowl. Whisk until combined. Slowly pour in the oil, whisking until emulsified.

3 Drizzle the dressing over the dandelion greens and toss to coat. Serve immediately as a side dish.

Other uses
❧ Make a brew of caffeine-free coffee using dried, roasted dandelion root.
❧ Fry cleaned dandelion flower tops and young leaves in batter to create crunchy fritters.

STYLE
BLOWBALL PAPERWEIGHT

Preserve a delicate dandelion seed ball in resin to enjoy the wonder of its construction year round.

Makes 1 paperweight
Dandelion clock (picked before opening)
Mould release spray
Dome-shaped mould approx. 8–10cm (3–4in) diameter
250ml (8oz) epoxy resin kit
2 plastic cups
Wooden spatula
Soft microfibre cloth

1 Pick a dandelion before it puffs and place in a jar. The clock should emerge within 1–2 days.

2 Wash and thoroughly dry the mould with a microfibre cloth. Place on a flat surface protected with wax paper. Spray inside the mould with release spray.

3 Wearing gloves, mix resin and catalyst according to the instructions on the box. Stir very gently to avoid bubbles. Carefully pour the resin into the mould.

4 Trim the dandelion clock stem (leave just enough to hold) and slowly push the seedhead into the resin – this may take a few minutes.

5 Leave to dry for the suggested time, usually around 72 hours.

6 Release the paperweight from the mould and buff with microfibre cloth.

7 If desired, mount on a dark background for contrast.

Other uses
❧ Offer guests dandelion-infused homemade lemonade, a non-alcoholic beverage best served in a Bohemian glass jug.
❧ Create lemon-yellow bars of soap, rich in dandelion-infused oil (see page 18) and cocoa butter.

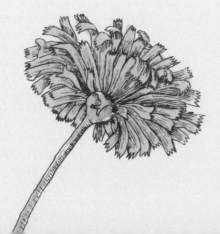

THYME
Thymus, Lamiaceae family

Tiny-leaved, aromatic, warmly pungent and antiseptic thyme (*Thymus*) has been cultivated since ancient times, certainly since the plant-inspired chronicles of Theophrastus, Dioscorides and Pliny. In these works, several species of this versatile herb are mentioned with obvious familiarity. Emblem of action, daring and courage – particularly during the Age of Chivalry (1100–1500) – favoured by fairies, a key component of *bouquet garni*, and an alluring and important source of nectar for bees, this is one herb that no garden, balcony or windowsill should be without.

❧ THE DESCRIPTION This evergreen, woody-based perennial has small aromatic leaves and whorls of small, tubular, purple, pink or white flowers. Common or garden thyme (*Thymus vulgaris* – pictured), wild or creeping thyme (*T. serpyllum*) and lemon thyme (*T. × citriodorus*) are among numerous varieties differentiated by leaf or flower colour, scent, flavour, habit or provenance.

❧ THE NAME One school of thought links the common name thyme and genus name *Thymus* to the ancient Greek word *thumus* or *thomus* signifying courage and in light of thyme's spiritual associations; another to the Greek word *thuo* meaning 'to fumigate' relating to the plant's aroma or use as incense. *Vulgaris* means a commonly found herb, while *serpyllum* refers to a creeping tendency and *citriodorus* to a lemon-like scent.

❧ THE PLACE Several species of *Thymus* are native to western Mediterranean regions including Greece, Italy and Spain but this ubiquitous plant's spread extends to many other temperate regions of Europe, North Africa and Asia. Its native habitat includes sandy-soiled heaths, rocky outcrops, hills and sandbanks. It thrives in well-drained soils in full sun and needs good drainage over winter.

❧ THE TIME Propagate by seed under cover in spring or by dividing plants or taking cuttings before flowering. Woody stemmed herbs such as thyme are also best harvested just before blooming to maintain flavour. Cut stems for drying just above a leaf node to encourage more foliage. Harvest the edible flowers in summer.

❧ THE VIRTUES Thyme 'purges the body of phlegm, and is an excellent remedy for shortness of breath' (Nicholas Culpeper, *Complete Herbal*, 1653). Now known to contain the naturally antibacterial and antiseptic phenol known as thymol, it is still used today to help ease coughs, congestion or a sore throat. Fresh or dried thyme is also delicious in roasts, biscuits, cakes, breads, vinegar and as syrup in drinks.

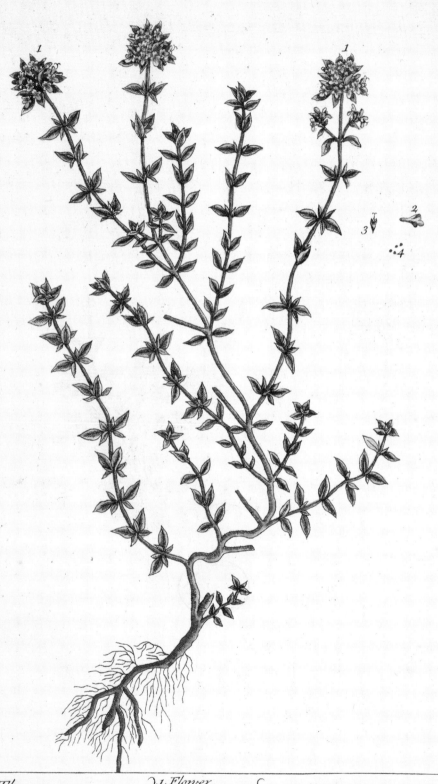

Plate 211.

Thyme.

1. *Flower.*
2. *Flower separate.*
3. *Calix.*
4. *Seed.*

Thymus.

Eliz. Blackwell delin. sculp. et Pinx.

HEAL
SORE THROAT SYRUP

Thyme has been used for thousands of years to help remedy sore throats and coughs, often delivered in the form of an infused tea, honey or syrup. Thyme syrup also adds a lovely herby twist to cocktails such as a gin and tonic or paired with grapefruit, vodka and lime.

Makes 1 x 500ml (17½ fl oz) jar
8 fresh thyme sprigs
10cm (4in) kitchen twine
250ml (¾ cups) honey (preferably raw and organic)

1 Secure the thyme sprigs into a bundle with the kitchen twine.

2 Combine 250ml (1 cup) of water and the honey in a pan. Bring to a gentle boil. Whisk until combined then turn off the heat.

3 Add the thyme to the honey syrup. Cover and let steep for 30 minutes.

4 Remove the thyme and discard in the compost. Strain the syrup through a fine mesh sieve into a sterilised 500ml (17½fl oz) glass lidded jar.

5 Seal and store in the fridge for up to 6 weeks and use as necessary.

Other uses
❧ Ease congestion with an inhalation of 1–2 tsp of dried thyme infused in a bowl of hot water.
❧ Boost energy and lift spirits by adding a few drops of thyme essential oil to a diffuser or oil burner.

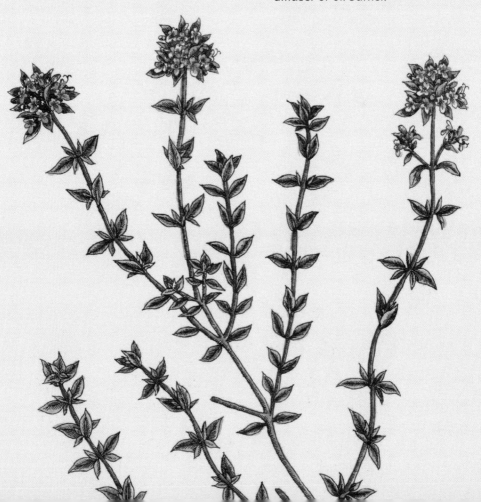

NOURISH THYME COMPOUND BUTTER

Mrs M. Grieve (*A Modern Herbal*, 1931) celebrates thyme 'for its use in flavouring stuffings, sauces, pickles, stews [and] soups'. It's also great in compound butter – delicious on cooked vegetables or muffins. Experiment with different varieties of thyme, or combine with garlic, lemon zest or other herbs such as rosemary or dill.

Makes 1 x 250g (9oz) butter roll
225g (1 cup) unsalted butter
1–2 tbsp fresh thyme leaves
Pinch of sea salt flakes (optional)

1 Cut the butter into cubes. Place in a bowl. Bring to room temperature.

2 Add the thyme leaves and salt flakes, if using, to taste. Beat with a stick blender until the butter is soft and the thyme mixed in well.

3 Shape the butter into a small log. Cover snugly with a reusable wax wrapper or baking paper. Chill in a fridge for at least 2 hours.

4 Store in the fridge or freeze. Serve up as a whole log of compound butter or slice into individual medallions.

Other uses
❧ Create a crunchy roasting crust of thyme leaves, breadcrumbs, paprika, garlic and olive oil.
❧ Try lemon thyme in shortbread or cookies for an earthy, tangy, sweet and savoury snack.

STYLE MIDSUMMER MINI-WREATH

Weave delicate midsummer wreaths of uplifting thyme to decorate a table setting, or for guests to take home. With its mats of tiny leaves, thyme was said to hide the tiny houses of fairy folk. The bower of the Fairy Queen Titania in William Shakespeare's *A Midsummer Night's Dream* (1595–96) was described as 'a bank where the wild thyme blows'.

Makes 1 wreath
Grapevine wire (steel wire in rustic twine)
Bunch of fresh thyme stems
Silver-coloured, thin floristry wire
Wire cutters

1 Create a 10cm (4in) hoop out of grapevine wire. Wrap the ends neatly.

2 Wind sprigs of thyme around the frame, attaching with small pieces of floristry wire if necessary.

3 Cover the whole hoop with thyme for a full wreath effect or just one side for a lovely asymmetrical effect. Or make a large version to wear as a crown.

Other uses
❧ Add a few drops of antibacterial and freshening thyme essential oil to a natural home-cleaning spray.
❧ Plant pots of flowering lemon thyme (*Thymus* × *citriodorus*) to attract bees by day and deter mosquitoes at dusk.

NETTLE
Urtica dioica, Urticaceae family

Ubiquitous stinging or common nettle (*Urtica dioica*) is often derided as a noxious weed, but this cucumber-spinach flavoured survivor has been a nutritional and medicinal mainstay in rural areas for centuries. The plant is native to Europe, much of temperate Asia, and western North Africa, and the strong inner fibres of its stalks were also used to make a type of ancient cloth. Samples have been found in European burial sites dating back to the Bronze Age. Stinging nettle was also introduced by settlers to North America, South America and Australia, where several subspecies now grow wild.

❧ **THE DESCRIPTION** 'Our common nettle' has 'heart-shaped, finely-toothed leaves tapering to a point' (Mrs M. Grieve, *A Modern Herbal*, 1931) with loose sprays of male flowers or more densely clustered female ones, both of a whitish-green hue but usually existing on separate plants. Most of the fibrous stem and leaf undersides are covered in downy stinging hairs, which produce irritating venom when pressed.

❧ **THE NAME** The genus name *Urtica* stems from the Latin for 'sting', *dioica* from the Greek for 'two houses' alluding to male and female flowers growing on separate plants. The canon of herbals is also rife with stinging nettle synonyms including the Greek *Akaluphe* (Dioscorides) and *Urtica vulgaris* (Nicholas Culpeper and Mrs M. Grieve). The name nettle is thought to stem from the Anglo-Saxon word *noedl* meaning needle.

❧ **THE PLACE** Legend has it that the Romans spread stinging nettles throughout Europe, flogging themselves with the skin-inflaming foliage to stay warm in winter. Plant remains from earlier archaeological sites, however, suggest that it was already a widespread European native. Nettle is a prolific, self-seeder so grow it by a compost heap (its nitrogen-rich leaves are a great compost accelerator) or forage for supplies.

❧ **THE TIME** Harvest young fresh nettle tops for culinary, medicinal or dyeing purposes in spring when plants are around 15–20cm (6–8in) high, or before they bloom (insoluble crystals of calcium carbonate are produced at flowering time) and wear gloves. To dry – useful for medicinal or cosmetic purposes – choose a fine, sunny morning, hanging bunches in a warm place.

❧ **THE VIRTUES** Stinging nettle, a traditional cure-all for everything from venomous bites to arthritis, is now known to be an antioxidant powerhouse of vitamins, minerals, protein and fatty acids. Access this goodness by eating nettle as a green vegetable or brewing into a tea (cooking or drying removes the sting). Naturally astringent, anti-inflammatory nettle can also help balance the complexion and ease aches and pains.

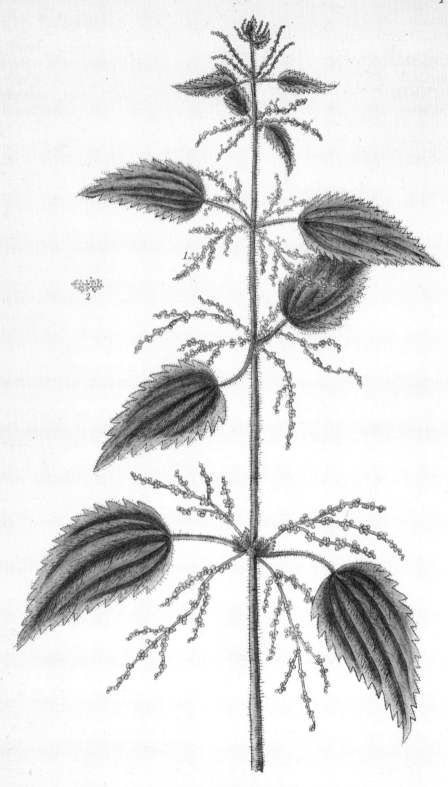

Plate 12.

Stinging Nettle

{ 1 *Flower* {
{ 2 *Seed* {

Urtica

Eliz. Blackwell delin. sculp. et Pinx.

HEAL
NETTLE TEA TONIC

Nettle provides rich pickings for a brew of immune-boosting tea, super high in vitamins A, B, C, D and K, flavonoids and minerals including potassium, magnesium, calcium and iron. Sip on up to four cups (250ml) a day as an anti-inflammatory, detoxifying tonic to help ease joint pain, urinary issues or skin problems.

Makes 4 cups
Small bunch (50g/2 cups) of fresh nettle leaves
2 tbsp honey

1 Wearing gloves, remove the tender nettle leaves from the main stalk. Leave as little stem as possible on each leaf.

2 Still wearing gloves, wash the leaves in warm water and then place in a large pan.

3 Add 1 litre (4 cups) of water and the honey. Bring to a boil then simmer for 15 minutes.

4 Strain immediately into cups and drink warm. Or decant into a teapot for drinking through the day. It's delicious cold with a slice of lemon or lime.

Other uses
❧ Infuse witch hazel extract with dried nettle leaves for 2 weeks, strain into a spray bottle and spritz onto face to help correct an oily complexion.
❧ Make an immune-boosting tincture by steeping dried nettle leaves in 80–90-proof vodka for around 2–3 weeks then decant into a dropper bottle to deliver 1–3 doses of 2–4ml (1/8oz) a day.

NOURISH
NETTLE SOUP

Swedish folk eat their blanched *nässelsoppa* (nettle soup) with sliced boiled egg, while one Native American recipe adds squash, and an Iranian dish involves chickpeas, lentils, turmeric powder and pomegranate molasses. Adapt the classic British recipe below to suit your taste.

Serves 4
150g (6 cups) fresh nettle leaves
1 white onion
450g (1lb) potatoes
60g (¼ cup) butter
1.5 litres (1½ quarts) vegetable stock
Sea salt and black pepper to taste
4 tbsp crème fraîche or yogurt, to serve
12 croutons, to serve (optional)
4 wild garlic flowers, to serve (optional)

1 Harvest tender nettle leaves before flowers emerge, wearing gloves to avoid stings. Carefully remove nettle leaves from the main stalk and wash.

2 Dice the onion and potatoes and cook gently in the butter in a large pan until soft.

3 Pour in the stock, bring to a boil, cover and then simmer for around 15 minutes.

4 Add the nettle leaves and simmer gently until tender (2–5 minutes at most).

5 Remove from the heat and leave to cool a little. Whizz into a purée with a stick blender.

6 Season with salt and pepper, then serve in bowls with a swirl of crème fraîche or yogurt, croutons and wild garlic flowers.

Other uses
❧ Make a tasty foraged pesto of blanched nettle leaves, wild garlic, hard cheese and breadcrumbs.
❧ Coat tender nettle leaves in batter, then deep fry into bite-sized fritters – frying takes the sting away.

STYLE
NETTLE DYE

Bright green nettle leaves produce a pale khaki, green or grey dye when applied to natural cloth or yarn, brightened by leaving the dye to steep for longer, or by pre-treating with an alum mordant or activating soya milk first. Nettles were used during the First World War to dye camouflage clothing and tents.

Makes 1 litre (1 quart)
Tote bag full of nettles (around 1kg/2lb 4 oz)
Piece of natural fabric, ribbon or yarn such
as cotton, linen, silk or wool, for dyeing

1 Harvest fresh nettles year-round, using gloves to avoid stings. Young fresh stems give the greenest hue. Remove bugs.

2 Chop the leaves and stalks. Place in a large, non-reactive pan – an aluminum pan can intensify the colour.

3 Cover with 1 litre (1 quart) of water and bring to a boil. Simmer gently for around an hour.

4 Remove from the heat and let the nettle leaves steep for 12 hours or overnight. Use tester strips to check hue. Strain out the nettle leaves when happy with the intensity. Have fun experimenting.

5 Place fabric, ribbon or yarn in the pan. Fully submerge with a wooden spoon. Simmer gently for an hour.

6 Remove from the heat. Leave to steep for 12 hours or overnight. Hang the fabric up to dry.

7 Rinse in warm water and dry again.

Other uses
❧ It's a painstaking business but the inner fibres (bast) of nettle stalks can be used to make paper as well as cloth.
❧ Combine dried nettle leaves, glycerine and aloe vera gel to make a clear, healing soap.

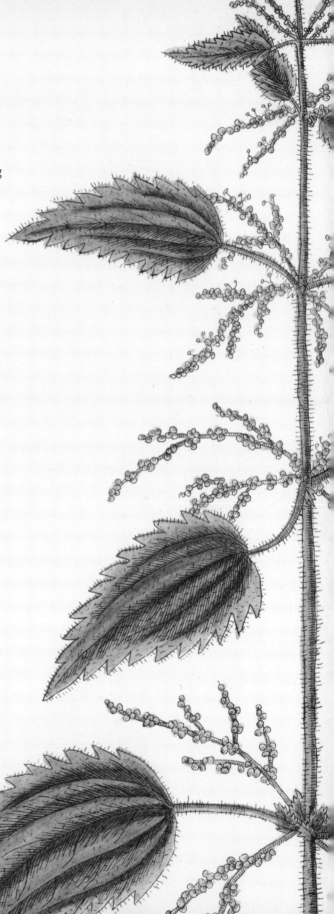

SWEET VIOLET
Viola odorata, Violaceae family

While John Gerard (*Herball*, 1597) describes a host of ancient violets in his rambling ode to this enigmatic little plant, Nicholas Culpeper (*Complete Herbal*, 1653) speaks only of '*Viola Odorata*' or 'sweet violet' – a sweet-scented, purple-flowered, creeping plant with heart-shaped leaves that has been cultivated for medicinal, culinary, fragrancing, cosmetic and symbolic purposes for hundreds of years. Sweet violet's delectable blooms – used by the Victorians as a token of love – are the source of its unique perfume as well as a deep violet colourant, and make a lovely garnish for desserts, salads or drinks. The leaves provide much of the plant's nutritional and therapeutic value.

❧ **THE DESCRIPTION** This hardy perennial with long-rooting runners forms a loose mat of dark green heart-shaped leaves in a basal rosette. The long-stalked aromatic flowers are usually dark purple but sometimes white. *Viola odorata* is one of several species thought to have been hybridised to produce the highly fragrant, single or double-flowered Parma violets such as 'Duchess de Parme'.

❧ **THE NAME** Elizabeth Blackwell illustrates a plant (see opposite) described as '*Viola Martia*' or 'March Violet' in *A Curious Herbal* (1737–39). While not accepted as a species name or synonym by botanists today, the illustration and description does fit with *Viola odorata* (sweet violet). The genus *Viola* stems from the Latin word for violet, while *odorata* alludes to sweet violet's elusive, sugary-sweet aroma and taste.

❧ **THE PLACE** Found near the edges of woods, in clearings, on hedge banks or as an uninvited guest of shaded lawn or gardens, *Viola odorata*'s native range extends across Europe to the Caucasus and to northwest Africa. It has also been introduced to and naturalised in swathes of North, South and Central America and Asia. Ideal in a rock garden or as ground cover, sweet violet flourishes in moist, well-drained soil in sun or partial shade.

❧ **THE TIME** Sweet violet displays its edible and medicinal foliage all year round; the scented flowers bloom over several weeks from late winter or early spring. Both can be harvested to use fresh or dried, making sure to choose an unpolluted patch of plants. Propagate by seed sown outdoors in autumn or divide established plants at that time.

❧ **THE VIRTUES** The 'flirty' scent of sweet violet comes from an alluring aromatic compound known as an ionone, which can switch scent receptors in the nose off and on again. The flowers add a deep violet colour to syrups and liqueurs, while the leaves are high in vitamins A and C and the compound rutin – an antioxidant, anti-inflammatory flavonoid that can help soothe thread veins, varicose veins, coughs or sunburn.

Plate 55.

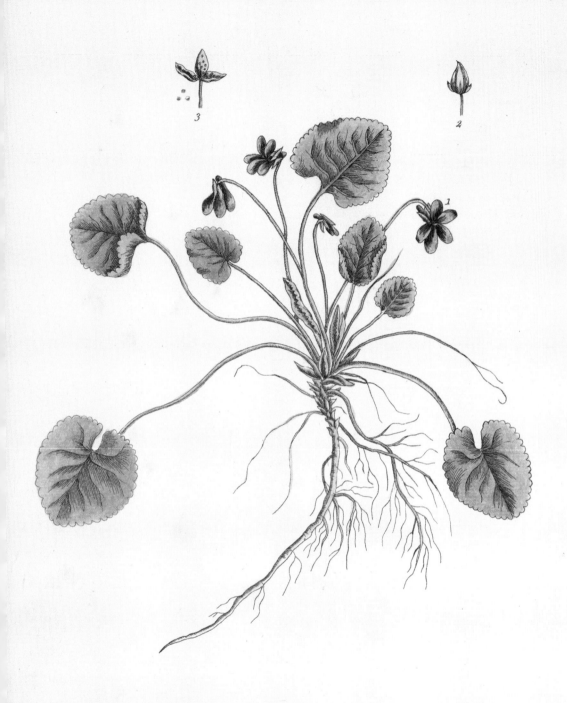

March Violet

Eliz Blackwell delin sculp et Pinx.

1 Flower
2 Fruit
3 Seed Vessell & Seed

Viola Martia

HEAL
VIOLET NIGHT CREAM

Combine naturally anti-inflammatory, sweet violet leaves and flowers with a moisturising carrier cream. Add vitamin E and sweet almond oil to make a nourishing night cream for the face, or a soothing balm for thread veins.

Makes 2 x 125ml (4fl oz) jars
2 handfuls of fresh violet flowers
6 violet leaves
250ml (1 cup) Paraben-free moisturising
   carrier cream
1 tbsp sweet almond oil
1 tbsp vitamin E or wheatgerm oil

1 Place the flowers, leaves and carrier cream in a bowl over a pan of boiling water.

2 Bring the water to a rolling boil then simmer for 20 minutes. Press the flowers and leaves into the cream with a wooden spoon to help infuse.

3 Remove the bowl from the heat. Let the cream cool for 10 minutes. Use a fine sieve to strain the cream into a mixing bowl.

4 Add the sweet almond oil and vitamin E or wheatgerm oil. Mix well.

5 Transfer the cream into 2 sterilised 125ml (4fl oz) lidded glass jars, and use a little each night or as required.

Other uses
❧ An infusion of violet leaves with or without flowers is a traditional remedy for coughs, sore throats, ulcers, headaches and insomnia.
❧ Blend a large handful of fresh violet petals with 125ml (½ cup) aloe vera gel to make a soothing gel for sunburn, insect bites or dry skin.

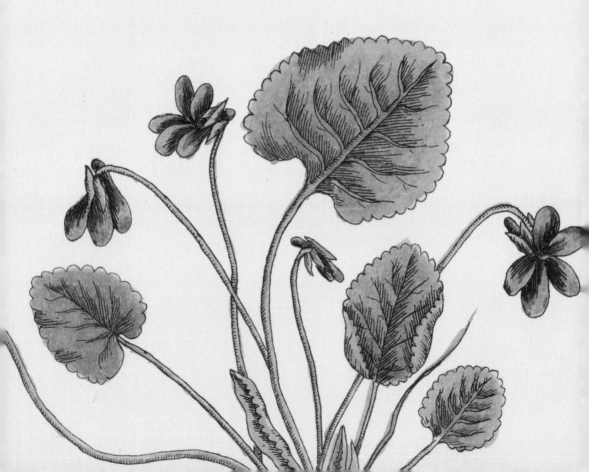

NOURISH
SWEET VIOLET SYRUP

Sweet violet syrup is one of the most traditional preparations of sweet violet flowers, it's subtle floral flavour and deep blue-purple hue adding a unique touch to a range of desserts and drinks. Mix with sparkling water or lemonade for a refreshing spring drink, add to buttercream or icing to decorate cakes or buns, or use in place of crème de violette in a deep purple Aviation cocktail.

Makes 1 x 250ml (8fl oz) jar
3–4 handfuls of fresh sweet violet flowers
150ml (2/3 cup) boiling water
300g (1½ cups) caster sugar

1 Remove and discard the green stalks and leaves from the flowers. Place the petals in a mixing bowl and cover with the boiling water. Place a clean cloth over the bowl. Leave to infuse for 24 hours.

2 Place another bowl over a pan of boiling water. Transfer the unstrained violet flower infusion into the bowl. Add the sugar and bring to a rolling boil. Stir until fully dissolved.

3 Strain the violet syrup through a fine sieve into a sterilised 250ml (8fl oz) airtight lidded glass jar. Store in a fridge for up to 12 months, and use as required.

Other uses
❧ Use naturally mucilaginous sweet violet leaves to thicken soups or stews, or scatter young leaves into salads.
❧ Use sweet violet flowers to decorate sweet or savoury dishes, either fresh or crystallised in a little egg white and sugar (see page 117).

STYLE
SWEET VIOLET PERFUME

It's notoriously hard to extract fresh sweet violet scent owing to the number of flowers and time required, but the experience of trying to capture just a tiny whiff of this enigmatic flower still feels magical.

Makes 250ml (8fl oz)
Several large handfuls of fresh violet flowers (picked regularly over the season)
250ml (1 cup) 80–90 per cent vodka
50ml (1¾fl oz) distilled water or sweet almond oil

1 Remove the stems and leaves from the flowers. Fill a 250ml (8fl oz) jar with petals. Don't pack too tightly.

2 Top up with vodka. Seal. Leave to infuse for 2–3 days until violet-scented and coloured.

3 Strain the liquid through muslin into a jug. Discard the flowers and pour the liquid back into the original jar.

4 Repeat the process for a few weeks or even months until the ensuing violet flower essence is deep purple and has the odour of violets. Store in the fridge.

5 To use as a perfume, half-fill a 100ml (3½fl oz) bottle with violet flower essence, top up with distilled water or sweet almond oil and apply to pulse points.

Other uses
❧ Present a partner or date with a Victorian-inspired romantic nosegay of scented sweet violets.
❧ Blend a large handful of sweet violet petals with 150g (¾ cup) coarse sea salt and 75g (heaped cup) Himalayan bath salts to make a soothing, violet-hued bath soak.

VIOLA HEARTSEASE
Viola tricolor, Violaceae family

The purple, yellow and white-petalled charming little herb and edible flower also known as heartsease shares the genus *Viola* with over 500 other species including sweet violet (*Viola odorata*, see page 154), European wild or field pansy (*V. arvensis*), the horned viola (*V. cornuta*) and its cultivated offspring, the large-flowered pansy (*V.* × *wittrockiana* hybrids). The mild-tasting flowers make a gorgeous garnish for sweet and savoury dishes, ices and drinks, and both leaves and flowers are traditional remedies for lung or heart ailments, skin conditions such as eczema, and infant fits and convulsions.

❀ **THE DESCRIPTION** Small, creeping viola heartsease sports a hairless stem flush with the soil, fine roots and mid-green, alternate, toothed and oval leaves. '*Viola tricolor*'s five-petalled flowers can vary in colour and size', the upper petals being the 'most showy in colour and purple in tint, while the lowest and broadest petal is usually a more or less deep tint of yellow' (Mrs M. Grieve, *A Modern Herbal*, 1931).

❀ **THE NAME** Heartsease, Jack-jump-up-and-kiss-me, Johnny-jump-up, love-in-idleness and kiss-her-in-the-buttery are just a few of the nicknames indicating the *Viola tricolor*'s past use in love potions. *Herba Trinitatis* (for its three-coloured or 'tricolor' flowers), the Anglo-Saxon *banewort* and the French *pensée* (a symbol of remembrance and Anglicised to pansy) are others. *Viola* is the Latin word for 'violet'.

❀ **THE PLACE** With a native range from Europe to Siberia to northwest Iran and introduced to much of North America, South America, Russia, parts of South Africa and southeast Asia, the humble *Viola tricolor* is ubiquitous as a 'wild pansy' as well as a cultivated ornamental or herb. Grow in any moderately fertile soil, in full sun or partial shade, in beds or pots. Avoid over-watering.

❀ **THE TIME** Viola heartsease can be grown as an annual, biennial or short-lived evergreen perennial. Sow seeds in autumn outdoors with some protection to germinate in spring. Leaves appear all year round but are best plucked in late summer. Blooms appear in spring, summer and autumn and should be picked when they have just opened. Deadhead regularly.

❀ **THE VIRTUES** Viola 'was, in the times of darkness, reckoned among the magic herbs' (Nicholas Culpeper, *The Complete Herbal*, 1653), harking back to the ancient Roman myth of Cupid turning the plant into a love potion with his arrow, or the Greek legend of Zeus feeding the flower to his secret lover Io. This pretty herb with edible flowers is still used to treat respiratory complaints and skin ailments.

Plate 44

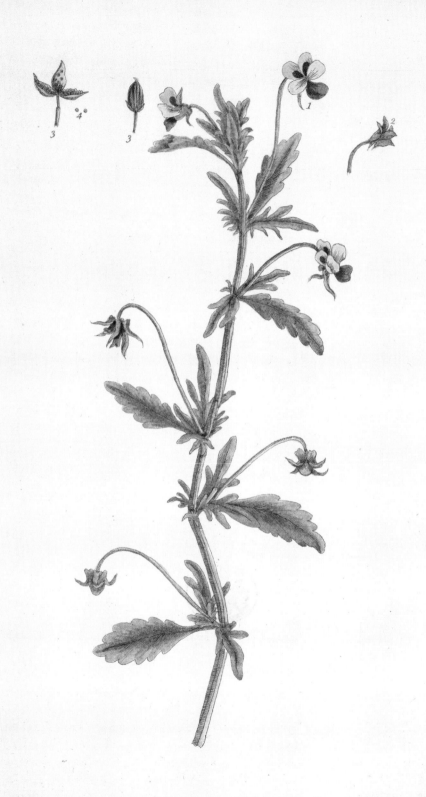

Heart's Eafe
Panfies

Eliz. Blackwell delin. sculp. et Pinx.

1 Flower
2 Flower Cup
3 Seed Veffell
4 Seed

Viola tricola

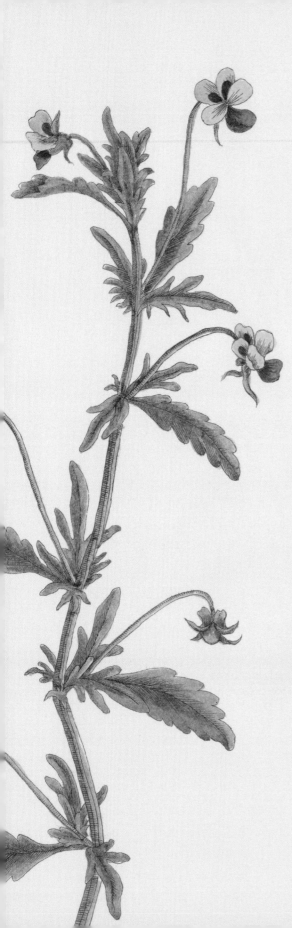

HEAL
HEARTSEASE TEA

While viola heartsease seeds and roots can be toxic, the edible flowers and leaves can be brewed into a flavonoid-rich tea to ease the heart by detoxifying, alleviating joint pain or relieving stress.

Makes 250ml (1 cup) tea
Large handful of fresh/dried viola heartsease flowers and leaves
250ml (1 cup) just-boiled water

1 Wash fresh flowers and leaves. Place on a baking tray. Leave to dry in the sun or in a warm place. Or source dried viola tea from a store.

2 Add 1 tbsp of dried flowers and leaves to the water. Leave to steep for 5–10 minutes to infuse.

3 Strain and drink in moderation – up to 3 cups a day for a limited time to avoid a laxative effect.

Other uses
❧ Make a poultice of naturally mucilaginous fresh or dried heartsease leaves, combined with honey, to help ease insect bites or stings.
❧ Blend a viola heartsease-chamomile flower infusion with beeswax, sweet almond oil, glycerine and emulsifying wax to make a soothing ointment for eczema or dry skin.

NOURISH
PRESSED VIOLA COOKIES

Bake gorgeous viola heartsease blooms directly onto cookies, adding a little egg white and sugar for sweetness and shine.

Makes around 30 cookies
225g (1 cup) unsalted butter, plus extra for greasing
240g (2 cups) plain flour, plus extra for dusting
100g (½ cup) lavender-infused sugar (see page 81) or caster sugar
Pinch of salt
1 tsp vanilla extract
Zest of 1 lemon
1 egg white, beaten
Around 30 fresh viola heartsease flowers
2 tbsp caster sugar

1 Preheat the oven to 180°C (350°F). Cut the butter into cubes. Cream until fluffy.

2 Fold in the flour, lavender sugar and pinch of salt. Add the vanilla extract and lemon zest. Beat into a soft dough.

3 Flour a clean surface. Roll the dough out to a 5mm (¼in) thickness. Cut into circles using a 5cm (2in) round cutter.

4 Grease a couple of large baking trays with butter. Arrange the circles 2.5cm (1in) apart. Bake for around 15 minutes or until light golden. Cool on wire racks.

5 Brush the top of each cookie with beaten egg white and place 1–2 flowers on top. Brush with egg white again. Sprinkle with caster sugar.

6 Return the cookies to the baking trays and bake for a further 5 minutes. Ensure edges do not burn. Cool on a wire rack.

Other uses
❀ Garnish spring salads, savoury and sweet canapés and cold seasonal soups with dainty viola heartsease flowers and leaves.
❀ Blitz a handful of well-washed tender leaves with 250ml (1 cup) of water to make a nourishing vitamin-C-rich distilled juice.

STYLE JOHNNY-JUMP-UP
ICE LOLLIES

Summer-blooming viola heartsease (Johnny-jump-up) flowers – or indeed other *Viola* species such as the horned pansy (*Viola cornuta*) or sweet violet (*V. odorata*, see page 154) – look delightful in ice cubes and ice lollies. Combine with coconut water, a squeeze of lime and a dash of honey to add a lovely refreshing flavour.

Makes 6–8 ice lollies
2 limes
500ml (2 cups) coconut water
2 tbsp honey
At least 30 edible *Viola* flowers
Flat silicone, 6–8-cavity ice-lolly mould (for easier arrangement)
6–8 ice-lolly sticks

1 Zest and juice the limes. Combine with the coconut water and honey in a jug and whisk.

2 Pour into the lolly mould. Use a toothpick to arrange viola flowers evenly in the juice.

3 Insert the lolly sticks. Freeze for several hours or overnight until hard.

4 To serve, run the mould under warm water for 30 seconds to help remove.

Other uses
❀ Viola heartsease is lovely grown between tiles, as a path edging or in pots or hanging baskets.
❀ Capture the beautiful colours and shapes of viola flowers using the hapa-zome method to press pigment print directly into paper or cloth as a nature-inspired artwork or textile design.

HERBARIUM

Design your own recipes and remedies to heal, nourish
and style with an at-a-glance herbarium of herbal virtues.

Herbs to Gather and Grow

❧ GARDEN ORNAMENTALS
Angelica
Calendula
Cornflower
Hyssop
Jasmine
Lavender
Liquorice
Lovage
Marjoram
Mint
Oregano
Parsley
Rose
Rosemary
Saffron
Sage
Salad burnet
Sorrel
Sweet cicely
Sweet violet
Thyme
Viola heartsease

❧ POLLINATOR FRIENDLY
Angelica
Borage
Chervil
Cornflower
Dandelion
Fennel
Hyssop
Lavender
Lemon balm
Marjoram
Rose
Rosemary
Saffron

Sage
Salad burnet
Sweet cicely
Sweet violet
Thyme
Viola heartsease

❧ WONDER WEEDS
Chicory
Dandelion
Nettle
Sorrel

❧ COMPANION PLANTING
Borage
Chervil
Cornflower
Parsley
Rose
Rosemary
Salad burnet
Sorrel
Sweet cicely
Sweet violet
Thyme
Viola heartsease

❧ TENDER HERBS
Basil
Chervil
Coriander
Fennel
Lemon balm
Mint
Parsley
Salad burnet
Sweet cicely
Viola heartsease

❧ BERRIES & SEEDS
Angelica
Elder
Fennel
Rose
Salad burnet

❧ GROUND COVER
Chamomile
Marjoram
Sweet violet
Thyme

❧ HEIGHT & STRUCTURE
Angelica
Elder
Fennel
Jasmine
Lavender
Liquorice
Lovage
Rose
Rosemary
Tarragon

❧ SUN LOVING
Basil
Borage
Calendula
Hyssop
Jasmine
Lavender
Lovage
Marjoram
Oregano
Sage
Tarragon
Thyme

❖ SHADE TOLERANT
Angelica
Coriander
Lemon Balm
Mint
Parsley
Salad burnet
Sorrel
Sweet cicely
Tarragon

❖ DROUGHT TOLERANT
Borage
Calendula
Lavender
Rosemary
Sage
Thyme

❖ EVERGREEN & SEMI-EVERGREEN
Hyssop (semi-evergreen)
Lavender
Marjoram
Oregano
(semi-evergreen)
Rose (semi-evergeen)
Rosemary
Sage
Thyme
Savory (winter; semi-evergreen)

❖ PERENNIAL
Angelica
Borage
Chamomile (Roman)
Fennel
Lavender
Lemon balm
Lovage
Mint
Salad burnet
Savory (winter)
Sorrel
Sweet violet

Tarragon
Viola heartsease (also annual)

❖ ANNUAL
Basil
Chamomile (German)
Chervil
Coriander
Savory (summer)

❖ FLOWERING
Angelica
Borage
Calendula
Chamomile
Chervil
Chicory
Cornflower
Dandelion
Elder
Fennel
Hyssop
Jasmine
Lavender
Lemon balm
Liquorice
Lovage
Marjoram
Mint
Oregano
Rose
Rosemary
Saffron
Sage
Salad burnet
Sweet cicely
Sweet violet
Thyme
Viola heartsease

❖ WINDOWSILLS & HOUSEPLANTS
Basil
Chervil
Mint

Oregano
Parsley
Rosemary
Thyme

❖ CONTAINER FRIENDLY
Basil
Borage
Calendula
Coriander
Lavender
Lemon balm
Mint
Oregano
Parsley
Rosemary
Sage
Sorrel
Sweet violet
Thyme
Viola heartsease

❖ GROW WITH CHILDREN
Basil
Calendula
Chamomile
Fennel
Lavender
Lemon balm
Mint
Sage
Thyme
Viola heartsease

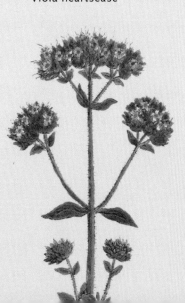

Herbs to Heal

❧ RELAXING
Lavender
Chamomile
Lemon balm
Fennel
Jasmine
Marjoram
Rose
Savory
Sweet violet

❧ CLEANSING
Chervil
Coriander
Dandelion
Fennel
Hyssop
Lavender
Mint
Nettle
Parsley
Sorrel

❧ UPLIFTING
Basil
Borage
Chamomile
Chervil
Lavender
Lemon balm
Marjoram
Mint
Rose
Rosemary
Saffron
Savory
Thyme

❧ BALANCING
Borage
Calendula
Chamomile
Fennel
Jasmine
Lavender

Lemon balm
Liquorice
Marjoram
Rose
Rosemary
Saffron
Sage
Salad burnet
Sweet violet

❧ COOLING
Coriander
Lavender
Lemon balm
Mint
Parsley
Rose
Salad burnet
Sweet violet

❧ ANTIOXIDANT
Basil
Calendula
Chervil
Coriander
Cornflower
Lemon balm
Marjoram
Nettle
Oregano
Parsley
Rose
Rosemary
Saffron
Sage
Salad burnet
Savory
Sorrel
Sweet cicely
Sweet violet
Thyme

❧ IMMUNE BOOSTING
Coriander
Elder

Mint
Nettle
Saffron
Salad burnet
Sorrel
Thyme

❧ ACHES & PAINS
Chamomile
Lavender
Marjoram
Mint
Nettle
Rose
Rosemary
Sage
Savory
Tarragon
Thyme

❧ SLEEP
Chamomile
Jasmine
Lavender
Marjoram
Savory
Sweet violet

❧ DIGESTIVE
Angelica
Chicory
Coriander
Fennel
Liquorice
Lovage
Mint
Oregano
Parsley
Rosemary
Sage
Salad burnet
Savory
Sorrel
Sweet cicely
Tarragon

✿ WOMEN'S HEALTH
Borage
Calendula
Fennel
Jasmine
Lavender
Rose
Sage

✿ CUTS & BRUISES
Calendula
Dandelion
Hyssop
Lemon balm
Salad burnet
Savory
Sweet cicely

✿ COUGHS & COLDS
Elder
Hyssop
Jasmine
Oregano
Sage
Savory
Sweet violet
Thyme

✿ SORE THROATS
Basil
Calendula
Chamomile
Elder
Hyssop
Liquorice
Mint
Oregano
Sage
Sweet violet
Thyme

✿ CIRCULATION
Angelica
Marjoram
Nettle

Rosemary
Sorrel
Sweet violet

✿ HEADACHES
Chamomile
Coriander
Lavender
Peppermint
Rosemary
Sweet violet

✿ SKIN TONICS
Borage
Calendula
Chamomile
Chervil
Cornflower
Dandelion
Jasmine
Lavender
Lemon balm
Nettle
Rose
Rosemary
Saffron
Sorrel
Sweet violet
Viola heartsease

✿ HAIR THERAPY
Jasmine
Lavender
Mint
Nettle
Rose
Rosemary

✿ FOCUS & MEMORY
Basil
Parsley
Rosemary
Saffron
Sage
Thyme

✿ ENERGY CLEARING
Angelica
Lavender
Rose
Rosemary
Sage
Thyme

✿ ANTI-BUG
Basil
Lavender
Lemon balm
Peppermint
Savory
Thyme

✿ TIRED FEET
Lavender
Lovage
Marjoram
Oregano

✿ CURE-ALL
Chamomile
Fennel
Lavender
Mint
Nettle
Rose
Rosemary

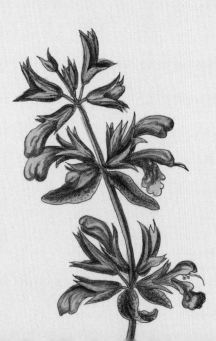

Herbs to Nourish

❧ AROMATIC
Angelica
Basil
Fennel
Hyssop
Lemon balm
Marjoram
Mint
Oregano
Rosemary
Sage
Savory
Sweet cicely
Tarragon
Thyme

❧ WARMING
Marjoram
Rosemary
Saffron
Sage
Savory
Tarragon
Thyme

❧ FLORAL
Elderflower
Jasmine
Rose
Sweet violet

❧ EDIBLE FLOWERS
Borage
Calendula
Chicory
Cornflower
Fennel
Lavender
Rose
Rosemary
Sweet cicely
Sweet violet
Viola heartsease

❧ FRUITS & SEEDS
Coriander
Elder
Fennel
Lovage
Oregano
Rose
Sweet cicely

❧ SWEET
Chervil
Chicory
Elderflower
Fennel
Jasmine
Lavender
Liquorice
Marjoram
Rose
Sweet cicely
Sweet violet
Tarragon

❧ BITTER
Chicory
Dandelion
Hyssop
Oregano
Rosemary
Savory

❧ EARTHY
Angelica
Coriander (seed)
Lovage
Marjoram
Oregano
Rosemary
Saffron
Sage
Savory
Tarragon
Thyme

❧ SOUR & CITRUS
Coriander
Lemon balm
Sorrel

❧ CAMPHOROUS
Oregano
Rosemary
Thyme

❧ FRESH
Chervil
Coriander
Fennel
Parsley
Salad burnet

❧ MINTY
Hyssop
Mint

❧ SEASONINGS & STUFFINGS
Hyssop
Marjoram
Oregano
Rosemary
Sage
Savory
Tarragon
Thyme

❧ INFUSIONS & COFFEE SUBSTITUTES
Chamomile
Chicory
Cornflower
Dandelion
Elderberry
Fennel
Jasmine
Lemon balm
Liquorice

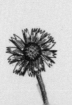

Mint
Nettle
Rose
Rosemary
Saffron
Sweet violet
Tarragon
Thyme

❀ SALADS
Basil
Borage
Calendula
Chamomile
Chervil
Chicory
Coriander
Dandelion
Fennel
Lovage
Mint
Parsley
Salad burnet
Sorrel
Sweet cicely
Sweet violet
Tarragon
Viola heartsease

❀ POTLETS, SOUPS & STEWS
Borage
Chervil
Coriander
Hyssop
Lovage
Nettle
Rosemary
Saffron
Savory
Sorrel
Sweet cicely
Sweet violet
Tarragon
Thyme
Viola heartsease

❀ SAUCES, PESTOS & DIPS
Basil
Chervil
Coriander
Hyssop
Marjoram
Mint
Nettle
Oregano
Parsley
Saffron
Salad burnet
Sorrel
Sweet cicely
Tarragon
Thyme

❀ PUDDINGS, PIES
& BAKES
Basil
Chervil
Elder
Fennel
Hyssop
Jasmine
Lavender
Liquorice
Oregano
Rose
Rosemary
Saffron
Savory
Sweet cicely
Sweet violet
Tarragon
Thyme

❀ FRITTERS
Borage
Dandelion
Elder
Fennel
Nettle
Sage
Sweet cicely

❀ ROBS & SYRUPS
Elder
Fennel
Lavender
Lovage
Rose
Saffron
Sweet cicely
Sweet violet
Thyme

❀ GARNISH
Borage
Calendula
Chamomile
Chervil
Coriander
Lavender
Lemon balm
Marjoram
Oregano
Parsley
Rose
Rosemary
Saffron
Sage
Salad burnet
Savory
Sweet cicely
Sweet violet
Tarragon
Thyme
Viola heartsease

❀ ROASTING
Hyssop
Lavender
Liquorice
Marjoram
Rosemary
Saffron
Sage
Savory
Tarragon
Thyme

Herbs to Style

❀ TABLE SETTING
Basil
Lavender
Marjoram
Mint
Oregano
Parsley
Rose
Rosemary
Sage
Sweet violet
Tarragon
Thyme
Viola heartsease

❀ PERFUME
Coriander
Fennel
Jasmine
Lavender
Marjoram
Rose
Sweet cicely
Sweet violet

❀ BOUQUETS
Calendula
Cornflower
Fennel
Lavender
Lemon balm
Mint
Rose
Rosemary
Sage
Sweet cicely
Sweet violet
Thyme
Viola heartsease

❀ CONFECTIONERY
Angelica
Fennel
Jasmine
Lavender

Liquorice
Lovage
Mint
Rose
Rosemary
Saffron
Sweet cicely
Sweet violet
Viola heartsease

❀ PRESSED BOTANICALS & JEWELLERY
Chervil
Cornflower
Fennel
Lavender
Lovage
Rose
Rosemary
Salad burnet
Sweet cicely
Sweet violet
Viola heartsease

❀ SCENTED CANDLES
Coriander
Fennel
Jasmine
Lavender
Lemon balm
Lovage
Mint
Rose
Rosemary
Sage
Sweet violet
Tarragon
Thyme

❀ HAIR GARLANDS
Calendula
Chamomile
Cornflower
Jasmine
Oregano

Rose
Rosemary
Thyme

❀ DRIED FLOWER WREATHS
Chamomile
Cornflower
Marjoram
Oregano
Rose
Rosemary
Thyme

❀ FLOWER CLOCKS
Calendula
Chicory
Dandelion
Jasmine
Rose

❀ COCKTAILS & LIQUEURS
Basil
Calendula
Chamomile
Lavender
Liquorice
Lovage
Mint
Oregano
Parsley
Rose
Rosemary
Saffron
Sage
Salad burnet
Savory
Sweet cicely
Sweet violet
Tarragon
Thyme
Viola heartsease

❀ CORDIALS & SOFT DRINKS
Chamomile
Dandelion

Elder
Lavender
Lovage
Mint
Rose
Sweet cicely
Sweet violet
Tarragon

❀ ICE CUBES & ICE LOLLIES
Borage
Calendula
Mint
Rose
Salad burnet
Sweet cicely
Sweet violet
Viola heartsease

❀ BATH SOAKS & SOAPS
Calendula
Cornflower
Dandelion
Fennel
Hyssop
Lavender
Lemon balm
Lovage
Marjoram
Mint
Nettle
Rose
Rosemary
Saffron
Sweet violet
Thyme

❀ NATURAL DYES & FOOD COLOURANTS
Calendula
Cornflower
Nettle
Rose
Saffron
Sweet violet

❀ OILS & VINEGARS
Calendula
Fennel (seed)
Rose
Rosemary
Saffron
Sage
Savory
Sweet cicely
Tarragon
Thyme
Viola heartsease

❀ HYDROSOLS & FLOWER WATERS
Calendula
Chamomile
Cornflower
Lavender
Lemon balm
Mint (spearmint)
Peppermint
Rose
Rosemary
Sage
Sweet violet
Thyme

❀ HOME CLEANING
Lavender
Rosemary
Sage
Sweet cicely
Thyme

❀ APRHRODISIAC & LOVE
Marjoram
Oregano
Rose
Saffron
Savory
Sweet violet
Tarragon

❀ WINE
Dandelion
Elder
Rose (hip)
Salad burnet

❀ KIDS' CRAFTING
Elder
Dandelion
Fennel
Lavender
Rose
Sweet violet
Thyme
Viola heartsease

❀ JUICES & SMOOTHIES
Coriander
Mint
Parsley
Salad burnet
Sorrel
Viola heartsease

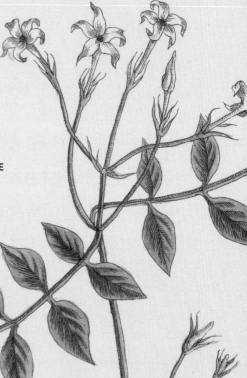

INDEX

(Page numbers in *italic* refer to illustrations, bold to recipes and remedies)

African marigold (*Tagetes*) 38
Age of Chivalry (1100–1500) 146
All's Well That Ends Well (Shakespeare) 102
American liquorice (*Glycyrrhiza lepidota*) 66
angelica (*Angelica archangelica*) 14, 20, 22–5, *23*, *24*, *25*
Angelica Jam 24
Angelica Root Tea 24
anise hyssop (*Agastache foeniculum*) 70
anise (*Pimpinella anisum*) 70
apple mint (*Mentha suaveolens*) 90
Arabian jasmine (*Jasminum sambac*) 74
Aromatic Pizza Sauce 109
Avicenna 10, 54, 78, 86

bachelor's buttons, *see* cornflower
Banks, Sir Joseph 13
basil (*Ocimum basilicum*) 17, 18, 21, 98–101, *99*, *101*
Béarnaise Sauce 33
Bee Kind Lip Balm 88
Belgian chicory (*Cichorium intybus* var. *foliosum*) 50
bergamot mint (*Mentha citrata*) 90
Blackrie, Elizabeth *see* Blackwell, Elizabeth
Blackwell, Alexander 8, 13
Blackwell, Elizabeth (née Blackrie) 7–13, 14, 46, 50, 58, 62, 66, 74, 78, 82, 94, 106, 114, 138, 154
Blair, Patrick 10
Blowball Paperweight **145**
blue bottle, *see* cornflower
Boerhaave, Herman 8
borage (*Borago officinalis*) 20, 34–7, *35*, *36*
Borage Leaf Ravioli **37**
Borage Seed Oil Soothing Facial Serum **36**
Botanicum Officinale (Miller) 9
A Box of *Fines Herbes* **29**
briar rose (*Rosa rubiginosa*) 114
British Pharmacopoeia (1864) 10
broad-leaved lavender 'Spica' (*Lavandula latifolia*) 78
Bronze Age 150
bronze-leaved fennel (*Foeniculum vulgare* 'Purpureum') 62
buckler leaf sorrel (*Rumex scutatus*) 122
bush basil (*Ocimum minimum*) 98

cabbage rose (*Rosa* × *centifolia*) 114
calendula (*Calendula officinalis*) *3*, 13, 18, 20, 38–41, *39*, *41*
Calendula Sunrise Soap **41**
Candied Lovage Stems **85**
Canon of Medicine (Avicenna) 10, 78, 86
Canterbury Tales (Chaucer) 66
caper plant (*Capparis spinosa*) 70
celery (*Apium graveolens*) 110

chamomile (*Chamaemelum nobile*) 13, 18, 20, 46–9, *47*, *48*
Chamomile Lawn **49**
Chaucer, Geoffrey 66
Chelsea Physic Garden 9
chervil (*Anthriscus cerefolium*) 19, 20, 26–9, *27*, *28*, *29*
Chervil Mayonnaise **28**
chicory (*Cichorium intybus*) 20, 50–3, *51*, *53*
Chicory Coffee **52**
Chicory O'clock **52**
Chimichurri Green Sauce **113**
Chinese *dong quai* (*Angelica sinensis*) 22
Chinese liquorice (*Glycyrrhiza uralensis*; *G. inflata*) 66
chives (*Allium schoenoprasum*) 16, 17
Chown, Vicky 10
clary sage (*Salvia sclarea*) 126
Classic Mojito **93**
Cleopatra 78
comfrey (*Symphytum*) 34
common elder (*Sambucus nigra*), *see* elder
common jasmine (*Jasminum officinale*), *see* jasmine
common mugwort (*Artemisia vulgaris*) 30
common nettle (*Urtica dioica*), *see* nettle
common sorrel (*Rumex acetosa*) 122
common thyme (*Thymus vulgaris*) 146, *147*, *148*
common wild marjoram, *see* oregano
Complete Herbal (Culpeper) 10, 22, 26, 38, 42, 46, 50, 74, 82, 90, 98, 106, 114, 122, 142, 146, 154, 158
Coriander and Pineapple Sorbet **57**
coriander (*Coriandrum sativum*) 16, 20, 54–7, *55*, *56*
corn mint (*Mentha arvensis*) 90
Cornflower Bath Bomb **45**
cornflower (*Centaurea cyanus*) *3*, 13, 19, 20, 42–5, *43*, *45*
cow parsley (*Anthriscus sylvestris*) 26, 94
creeping savory (*Satureja spicigera*) 138
creeping thyme (*Thymus serpyllum*) 146
Crystallised Rose Petals **117**
Culpeper, Nicholas 10, 14, 22, 26, 38, 42, 46, 50, 66, 74, 82, 90, 98, 102, 106, 114, 122, 142, 146, 150, 154, 158
A Curious Herbal (Blackwell) 7, 9, 10, 13, 46, 50, 58, 62, 78, 82, 94, 106, 114, 138, 154
curly parsley (*Petroselinum crispum*), *see* parsley

damask rose (*Rosa* × *damascena*) 114, *115*, *116*
Dandelion Salad **145**
dandelion (*Taraxacum officinale*) 21, 142–5, *143*, *144–5*
Dandelion Wine **144**
De Materia Medica (Dioscorides) 10, 66, 82, 90, 102, 114, 118, 134
Di Yu, *see* salad burnet
Digestive Tarragon Tea **32**
Dioscorides 10, 54, 62, 82, 90, 102, 106, 114, 118, 134, 146, 150
dog rose (*Rosa canina*) 114, 117
Drakenstein, Hendrik van Rheede tot 10

Earl Blue Tea **44**
Earth-Apple Porridge **49**
elder (*Sambucus nigra*) 19, 21, 130–3, *131, 132*
Elderberry Jelly **133**
Elderberry Rob Syrup **132**
Elderflower Cordial **133**
English lavender (*Lavandula angustifolia*) 78, 79
The English Physician Enlarged (Culpeper) 10
European liquorice (*Glycyrrhiza glabra*), *see* liquorice
European wild pansy (*Viola arvensis*) 158

false chamomile (*Matricaria chamomilla*) 46
Fave e Cicoria **52**
Fennel and Grapefruit Body Wash **65**
Fennel Breath Freshener **64**
fennel (*Foeniculum vulgare*) 13, 20, 62–5, *63, 64*
Fennel Fritters **65**
field marjoram (*Origanum vulgare*), *see* oregano
field pansy (*Viola arvensis*) 158
Finocchio (*Foeniculum vulgare* var. *dulce*) 62
First-aid Poultice **136**
flat-leafed parsley (*Petroselinum crispum*), *see* parsley
Florence fennel (*Foeniculum vulgare* var. *dulce*) 62
flower clocks 52
Focaccia di Genova **120–1**
forget-me-not (*Myosotis*) 34
Fowler, Alys 10
French lavender (*Lavandula stoechas*) 4, 5, 78, 80
French marigold (*Tagetes*) 38
French parsley (*Petroselinum crispum* 'French') 110
French sorrel (*Rumex scutatus*) 122
French tarragon (*Artemisia dracunculus* var. *sativa*) 30

garden basil (*Ocimum basilicum*), *see* basil
garden chicory (*Cichorium intybus*), *see* chicory
garden fennel (*Foeniculum vulgare*), *see* fennel
Garden Gimlet **137**
garden mint (*Mentha spicata*) 90
garden sorrel (*Rumex acetosa*) 122
garden thyme (*Thymus vulgaris*) 146, *147, 148*
The Gardener's Dictionary (Miller) 9, 62
garlic (*Allium sativum*; *A. sativum*) 145
General Historie of Plants (Gerard) 10
George III 13
Gerard, John 10, 14, 22, 26, 30, 34, 38, 46, 54, 58, 66,
    74, 82, 86, 102, 106, 118, 122, 130, 154
German chamomile (*Matricaria chamomilla*) 46
Gilded Rosemary Lollipops **121**
great burnet (*Sanguisorba officinalis*) 134
Greek oregano (*Origanum vulgare* subsp. *hirtum*)
    106
Greek sage (*Salvia fruticosa*) 126
green alkanet (*Pentaglottis sempervirens*) 34
Green Sauce **57**
Grieve, Mrs M. 10, 22, 30, 34, 38, 42, 46, 50, 54, 66,

70, 82, 86, 90, 94, 98, 110, 114, 117, 118, 126, 130, 134,
    142, 149, 150, 158

Hamburg parsley (*Petroselinum* var. *tuberosum*) 110
The Handmade Apothecary (Walker, Chown) 10
Happy Feet Oil **108**
Harding, Samuel 9, 13
hardneck garlic (*Allium sativum*) 145
Head-easing Steam **100**
Heartsease Tea **160**
hedgehog liquorice (*Glycyrrhiza echinata*) 66
hemlock (*Conium maculatum*) 22, 26, 94
Herb of Joy Cake **109**
Herb of Joy Vinegar **28**
Herbal Decoction **18**
Herbal Infused Oil **18–19**
Herbal Infused Syrup **19**
Herbal Infusion **18**
Herball (Gerard) 10, 22, 26, 30, 34, 38, 54, 58, 82, 86,
    118, 122, 130, 154
Herbes de Provence **140–1**
Historia Plantarum (Theophrastus) 10
holy basil (*Ocimum tenuiflorum*) 98
horned viola/pansy (*Viola cornuta*) 158, 161
Horologium Florae 52
horse mint (*Mentha longifolia*) 90
Hortus Indicus Malabaricus (Drakenstein) 10
Hyssop-glazed Carrots **73**
hyssop (*Hyssopus officinalis*) 19, 20, 70–3, *71, 72*
Hyssop Oxymel **72**
Hyssop Ritual Bath **73**

infused rose oil (*oleum rosaceum*) 114
Invigorating Hair Rinse **120**
Isabella, or The Pot of Basil (Keats) 98
Italian parsley (*Petroselinum crispum* var. *neopolitanum*)
    110

Jasmine Body Butter **76**
jasmine (*Jasminum officinale*) 18, 20, 74–7, *75, 77*
Jasmine Tea **76**
Johnny-Jump-Up Ice Lollies **161**

Kahwa Tea **60**
Keats, John 98
Kombucha **96**

large-flowered pansy (*Viola* × *wittrockiana* hybrids) 158
Lavender Dream Pillow **81**
Lavender Healing Salve **80**
lavender (*Lavendula*) 4, 13, 15, 16, 18, 19, 20, 78–81,
    79, 80
Lavender Sugar **81**
Lemon and Coriander Soup **56**
Lemon Balm Bouquet **89**

171

Lemon Balm Iced Tea **89**
lemon balm (*Melissa officinalis*) 18, 21, 86–9, *87*, *88*
lemon basil (*Ocimum × citriodorum*) 98
lemon thyme (*Thymus × citriodorus*) 146
Leyel, Hilda 10
Libanotis coronaria 118
Linnaeus, Carl 13, 46, 50, 52, 106
Liquorice Candy **69**
Liquorice Energy Balls **69**
liquorice (*Glycyrrhiza glabra*) 20, 66–9, *67*, *68*
Liquorice Toothbrush **68**
London Pharmacopoeia (1618) 10
Lovage and Potato Soup **84**
lovage (*Levisticum officinale*) 20, 82–5, *83*, *84*, *85*
Love Potion **141**

Marathokeftedes **65**
Marischal College, Aberdeen 8
marjoram 19
marjoram (*Origanum majorana*) 16, 21, 102–5, *103*, *104*
marsh selinon (*Heleioselinon*; *Eleioselinon*) 110
De Materia Medica (Dioscorides), *see De Materia Medica*
Mead, Dr Richard 9
meadow saffron (*Colchicum autumnale*) 58
Medical Botany (Woodville) 10
Mexican tarragon (*Tagetes lucida*) 30
Midsummer Mini-wreath **149**
A Midsummer Night's Dream (Shakespeare) 149
Miller, Joseph 10
Miller, Philip 9, 62
The Miller's Tale (Chaucer) 66
mint (*Mentha*) 17, 18, 21, 90–3, *91*, *92–3*
A Modern Herbal (Fowler) 10
A Modern Herbal (Grieve) 10, 22, 30, 34, 38, 42, 46, 50, 54, 66, 70, 82, 86, 90, 94, 98, 110, 114, 117, 118, 126, 130, 134, 142, 149, 150, 158
Mojito **93**
Mojo Verde **57**
Moroccan Mint Tea **92**
Mukhwas **64**
Muscle Relief Massage Oil **104**

narrow-leaved 'Lavandula' (*Lavandula angustifolia*) 78
Natural Bite Relief **140**
Naturalis Historia (Pliny) 10, 90, 110, 118
Nettle Dye **153**
Nettle Soup **152**
Nettle Tea Tonic **152**
nettle (*Urtica dioica*) 16, 18, 21, 150–3, *151*, *153*
Nourse, John 9, 13

orange mint (*Mentha citrata*) 90
oregano (*Origanum vulgare*) 16, 18, 21, 102, 106–9, *107*, *108*

Paradisi in Sole, Paradisus Terrestris (Parkinson) 10, 22, 86
Parkinson, John 10, 14, 22, 66, 86, 142
Parma violets, *see* sweet violet
Parsley Detox Juice **112**
parsley (*Petroselinum crispum*) 16, 21, 26, 110–13, *111*, *113*
parsnip-rooted Hamburg parsley (*Petroselinum* var. *tuberosum*) 110
Pea and Mint Soup **92**
pennyroyal (*Mentha pulegium*) 90
peppermint (*Mentha × piperita*) 18, *18,* 90
Persephone 90
Persian Jewelled Rice **60**
Pesto alla Genovese **100**
Pharmaco-Botanologia (Blair) 9
Philosophia Botanica (Linnaeus) 52
pineapple mint (*Mentha suaveolens*) 90
pink-flowered savory (*Satureja thymbra*) 138
pink hyssop (*Hyssopus officinalis* 'Roseus') 70
Pliny the Elder 10, 50, 54, 62, 86, 90, 106, 110, 118, 146
pot marjoram (*Origanum onites*) 102
Pressed Viola Cookies **161**
Provence rose (*Rosa × centifolia*) 114
Purifying Smoke Stick **129**
purple sage (*Salvia officinalis* 'Purpurascens') 126

radicchio (*Cichorium intybus* var. *foliosum*) 50
Rainbow Flower Summer Rolls **40**
Rand, Isaac 9
red chicory (*Cichorium intybus*) 50
red rose (*Rosa gallica*) 114
Rhodon, see rose
rock rose (*Cistus ladanifer*) 13
rock selinon (*Oreoselinon*; *Petroselinon*) 110
Roman chamomile (*Chamaemelum nobile*), *see* chamomile
Roman Empire 150
Rose Hip Syrup **117**
rose (*Rosa*) 13, 18, 19, 21, 114–17, *115*, *116*
Rose Water Hydrosol **116**
Rosemary Focaccia **120–1**
Rosemary Gladstar's Herbal Recipes for Vibrant Health (Leyel) 10
Rosemary Lollipops **121**
rosemary (*Rosmarinus officinalis*) 13, 16, 18, 21, 118–21, *119*, *120*
Royal College of Physicians 10
Royal Society of London 13
Russian tarragon (*Artemisia dracunculus dracunculus* var. *inodora*; *A. dracunculoides*) 30

saffron (*Crocus sativus*) 13, 19, 20, 58–61, *59*, *61*
Saffron Negroni **61**
Sage and Onion Stuffing **129**
Sage Hot-flush Tincture **128**

sage (*Salvia officinalis*) 13, 16, 18, 19, 21, 126–9, *127, 129*
salad burnet (*Sanguisorba minor*) 21, 134–7, *135, 136*
Salad Burnet Vinegar and Vinaigrette **137**
Savory Love Potion **141**
savory (*Satureja*) 21, 138–41, *139, 140–1*
Scandix cerefolium, see chervil
Sensual Candle **77**
Shakespeare, William 102, 149
sheep's sorrel (*Rumex acetosella*) 122
Sicilian sumac (*Rhus coriaria*) 105
Skin-calming Foot Soak **84**
Skin-Soothing Bath Soak **40**
Sleep-easy Linen Spray **105**
Sloane, Sir Hans 9
Smedley, Anne Constance 9
Society of Apothecaries 9
Soothe-Me Chamomile Tea **48**
Soothing Mister **44**
Sore Throat Syrup **148**
sorrel (*Rumex*) 21, 122–5, *123, 125*
Sorrel Sauce **124**
Sorrel Smoothie **125**
Sorrel Soup **124**
Sowerby, James 10
Spanish jasmine (*Jasminum grandiflorum*) 74
spearmint (*Mentha spicata*) 90
species parsley (*Petroselinum crispum*), see parsley
Species Plantarum (Linnaeus) 13, 50
spike lavender (*Lavandula latifolia*) 78
Starflower Pimm's **37**
summer savory (*Satureja hortensis*) 138
Sweden, King of 13
Sweet Basil Flower Oil **101**
sweet basil (*Ocimum basilicum*), see basil
sweet briar rose (*rosa rubiginosa*) 114
Sweet Cicely and Rhubarb Compote **97**
Sweet Cicely Kombucha **96**
sweet cicely (*Myrrhis odorata*) 21, 26, 94–7, *95, 96*
Sweet Cicely Schnapps **97**
sweet marjoram (*Origanum majorana*), see marjoram
Sweet Violet Perfume **157**
Sweet Violet Syrup **157**
sweet violet (*Viola odorata*) 19, 21, 154–7, *155, 156*, 158, 161
Syrian oregano (*Origanum syriacum*) 70

Tabboulleh **112**
Tang Materia Medica (659 BC) 142
Tarkhun **33**
tarragon (*Artemisia dracunculus*) 16, 17, 18, 19, 20, 30–3, *31, 32*
Tarragon-ade **33**
Thai basil (*Ocimum basilicum* var. *thyrsiflora*) 98
Theatrum Botanicum (Parkinson) 142
Theophrastus 10, 54, 62, 110, 114, 146

Thyme Compound Butter **149**
thyme (*Thymus*) 13, 16, 18, 19, 21, 146–9, *147, 148*
toxic hemlock (*Conium maculatum*) 22, 26, 94
true chamomile (*Chamaemelum nobile*), see chamomile
true endive (*Cichorium endivia*) 50
true hyssop (*Hyssopus officinalis*), see hyssop
true saffron (*Crocus sativus*), see saffron
true tarragon (*Artemisia dracunculus* var. *sativa*) 30
tuft-flowered lavender 'Stoechas' (*Lavandula stoechas*) 78
Turky balm, see lemon balm
Turning the Pages™ 13
Tutti Frutti Ice Cream **25**

valerian (*Valeriana officinalis*) *10, 11*
variegated sage (*Salvia officinalis* 'Tricolor') 126
Viola Cookies **161**
viola heartsease (*Viola tricolor*) 14, 18, 21, 158–61, *159*, 160
Violet Night Cream **156**

Walker, Kim 10
water mint (*Mentha aquatica*) 90
white hyssop (*Hyssopus officinalis* f. *albus*) 70
white rose (*Rosa alba*) 114
wild angelica (*Angelica sylvestris*) 22
wild chicory (*Cichorium intybus*), see chicory
wild coriander (*Coriandrum tordylium*), see coriander
wild crocus (*Crocus cartwrightianus*) 58
wild fennel (*Foeniculum vulgare*), see fennel
wild garlic (*Allium ursinum*) 145
wild marjoram (*Origanum vulgare*), see oregano
wild mint (*Mentha longifolia*) 90
wild pansy (*Viola arvensis*) 158
wild parsley (*Petroselinum crispum*), see parsley
wild rose (*Rosa*) 12, 13, 114
wild saffron (*Colchicum autumnale*) 58
wild succory (*Cichorium sylvestre*) 50
wild thyme (*Thymus serpyllum*) 146
winter jasmine (*Jasminum nudiflorum*) 74
winter marjoram (*Origanum vulgare* var. *hirtum*) 102
winter savory (*Satureja montana*) 138
witloof (*Cichorium intybus* var. *foliosum*) 50
wood sorrel (*Oxalis acetosella*) 122
Woodville, William 10
wormwood (*Artemisia absinthium*) 30

yarrow (*Achilea millefolium*) 17
yellow-leaved sage (*Salvia officinalis* 'Aurea') 126

Za'atar Spice Mix **105**
Zesty Dandelion Salad **145**
Zeus 90, 158

RESOURCES

BIBLIOGRAPHY

The following (chronological) list of original herbals, amended or enlarged versions and modern-English translations includes titles available via the British Library catalogue with options to view online via resources such as British Library Turning the Pages system, biodiversitylibrary.org and archive.org. With thanks to all those who have laboured with passion and purpose over the centuries to keep such crucial knowledge alive.

Theophrastus, *Historia Plantarum* (350–287 BC)
Theophrastus, Enquiry into plants and minor works on odours and weather signs, with an English translation by Sir Arthur Hort, Bart., M. A. (London, William Heinemann London; New York, G. P. Putnam's Sons, 1916)
Available online at www.biodiversitylibrary.org// bibliography/24769#/summary

Dioscorides, *De Materia Medica* (AD 50–70)
De materia medica by Pedanius Dioscorides of Anazarbus, translated by Lily Y. Beck (Hildesheim: Olms-Weidmann, 2017)

Dioscorides, *De materia medica*, translated by Tess Anne Osbaldeston as *The Herbal of Dioscorides the Greek* (Ibidis Press, South Africa, 2000)
Available online at archive.org/details/de-materia-medica/page/n2

Pliny (the Elder), *Naturalis Historia* (AD 77–79)
Natural history of Pliny, translated with copious notes and illustrations, by the late John Bostock and H. T. Riley (H. G. Bohn, London, 1855–57)
Available online at www.biodiversitylibrary.org// bibliography/8126#/summary

Avicenna, *Canon of Medicine* (1025)
A Treatise on the Canon of Medicine of Avicenna incorporating a translation of the first book, By O. Cameron Gruner (Luzac & Co, London, 1930; AMS Press, New York, 1973)
Available online at archive.org/stream/ AvicennasCanonOfMedicine/9670940-Canon-of-Medicine_djvu.txt

John Gerard, *Herball* (1597)
Herball, or, Generall historie of plantes /gathered by John Gerarde of London, master in chirurgerie (John Norton, London, 1597)
Available online at www.biodiversitylibrary.org// bibliography/51606#/summary

Herball, or, Generall historie of plantes /gathered by John Gerarde of London master in *chirurgerie;* very much

enlarged and amended by Thomas Johnson citizen and apothecarye of London (Adam Islip, Joice Norton and Richard Whitakers, London, 1636)
Available online at https://www.biodiversitylibrary.org// bibliography/8044#/summary

John Parkinson, *Paradisi in Sole, Paradisus Terrestris* (1629) & *Theatrum Botanicum* (1640)
Paradisi in Sole, Paradisus Terrestris. Or A Garden of ... flowers; ... with a Kitchen garden ... and an Orchard; together with the right orderinge, planting and preserving of them and their uses and vertues, etc. [With woodcuts.] by John Parkinson (H. Lownes and R. Young, London, 1629). Available online at www.biodiversitylibrary.org/ bibliography/118671#/summary

Theatrum Botanicum: The Theater of Plants, or, an Herball of large extent, etc. by John Parkinson (T. Cotes, London, 1640)
Available online at www.biodiversitylibrary.org/ bibliography/152383#/summary

Nicholas Culpeper, *The English Physician, etc. / Complete Herbal* (1653)
The English physician, etc. by Nicholas Culpeper (Peter Cole, London, 1653)

The complete herbal; to which is now added, upwards of one hundred additional herbs, with a display of their medicinal and occult qualities ... to which are now first annexed, The English physician, enlarged, and Key to physic ... New edition ... Illustrated by engravings of numerous British herbs and plants, correctly coloured from nature. by Nicholas Culpeper (Thomas Kelly & Co., London, 1863). Available online at http://access.bl.uk/item/viewer/ark:/81055/vdc_100025476968.0 x000001#?c=0&m=0&s=0&cv=292&xywh=-1%2C-3735%2C4930%2C10854

Elizabeth Blackwell, *A Curious Herbal* (1737–39)
A curious herbal :containing five hundred cuts, of the most useful plants, which are now used in the practice of physick engraved on folio copper plates, after drawings taken from the life by Elizabeth Blackwell (Samuel Harding, London, 1737–39). Available online at www.biodiversitylibrary.org/bibliography/571#/summary
Available online at www.bl.uk/turning-the-pages/?id=635a7cc0-a675-11db-a027-0050c2490048&type=book

Carl Linnaeus, *Species Plantarum* (1753)
Species plantarum / [by] C. Linnaeus, a Ray Society facsimile of the edition of 1753 with an introduction by W. T. Stearn and an appendix by J. L. Heller (London, 1957–59)

Mrs M. Grieve, *A Modern Herbal* (1931)
A modern herbal : the medicinal, culinary, cosmetic and economic properties, cultivation and folklore of herbs, grasses, fungi, shrubs and trees with all their modern scientific uses / by Mrs M. Grieve; edited and introduced by Mrs C.F. Leyel. (Jonathan Cape, London, 1974). Available online at www.botanical.com/botanical/ mgmh/mgmh.html

WEBSITES

Globally accepted, up-to-date resources relating to the naming, description, provenance, and cultivation of herbs and other plants.

Kew Plants of the World Online
   www.plantsoftheworldonline.org/
Royal Horticultural Society (RHS) www.rhs.org.uk/Plants
The Plant List www.theplantlist.org/

ELIZABETH BLACKWELL

Articles and other works specifically relating to the life and works of author and illustrator Elizabeth Blackwell (1707–1758) and her *A Curious Herbal* (1737–39).

The Curious Herbal, etc. by Anna Constance Smedley (London, New York, 1930)
A Curious Herbal by British Library Collections (date not specified)
www.bl.uk/collection-items/a-curious-herbal-dande
   lion?gclid=CjwKCAiA8K7uBRBBEiwACOm4d5atTp
   cCGSWomVgMn8DhI3kBBEdele7AskQpYCGzja3_
   NDfaG9v53RoC_z0QAvD_BwE
Elizabeth Blackwell – the forgotten herbalist by Madge Bruce, Wiley Online Library (2003)
onlinelibrary.wiley.com/doi/full/10.1046/j.1471-
   1842.2001.00330.x
Elizabeth Blackwell by Huber M. Walsh, Missouri Botanical Gardens Library (date not specified)
www.illustratedgarden.org/mobot/rarebooks/author.
   asp?creator=Blackwell,%20Elizabeth&creatorID=68
Elizabeth Blackwell by National Library of Scotland (date not specified)
www.nls.uk/learning-zone/science-and-technology/
   women-scientists/elizabeth-blackwell
Will the real Elizabeth Blackwell please stand up by New York Botanical Garden Plant Talk (2013)
www.nybg.org/blogs/plant-talk/2013/07/exhibit-news/
   will-the-real-elizabeth-blackwell-please-stand-
   up/#more-37867
About Elizabeth Blackwell, by Botanical Art & Artists (date not specified)
www.botanicalartandartists.com/about-elizabeth-
   blackwell.html

FURTHER READING

The Heritage Herbal offers an introduction to using herbs to heal, nourish and style. For more in-depth advice, inspiration on growing and gathering, foraging and wild food, herbs and herbal preparations and aromatherapy the following titles are recommended.

A Modern Herbal by Alys Fowler (Michael Joseph, 2019)
Food for Free by Richard Mabey (Collins, 2012)
Foraging & Feasting: A Field Guide and Wild Food Cookbook by Dina Falconi and Wendy Hollender (Botanical Arts Press LLC, 2013)
Jekka's Herb Cookbook by Jecca McVicar (Firefly Books, 2012)
Rosemary Gladstar's Herbal Recipes for Vibrant Health by Rosemary Gladstar (Storey Publishing, 2008)
Rosemary Gladstar's Medicinal Herbs: A Beginner's Guide by Rosemary Gladstar (Storey Publishing, 2012)
The Complete Aromatherapy and Essential Oils Sourcebook by Julia Lawless (Sterling, 2018)
The Eatweeds Cookbook by Robin Harford (Eatweeds, 2015)
The Edible City: A Year of Wild Food by John Rensten (Boxtree, 2016)
The Encyclopedia of Essential Oils by Julia Lawless (Conari Press, 2014)
The Gardener's Companion to Medicinal Plants by Royal Botanic Gardens Kew and Jason Irving (Frances Lincoln, 2017)
The Handmade Apothecary by Vicky Chown and Kim Walker (Kyle Books, 2017)
The Herbal Remedy Handbook by Vicky Chown and Kim Walker (Kyle Books, 2019)
The Illustrated Herbal Handbook by Juliette de Bairacli Levy (Faber & Faber, 1982)
The New Wildcrafted Cuisine by Pascal Bauder (Chelsea Green Publishing Co. 2016)
Wild Food by Roger Phillips (Pan Books, 1983; Macmillan 2014)

INGREDIENTS

Many ingredients in the recipes and remedies of this book can be sourced from the garden, in the wild or in a local store or supermarket. Where specialist items such as dried herbs, essential oils and cosmetic bases are required, please source as sustainably as possible from a responsible provider.

Aqua Oleum www.aqua-oleum.co.uk
G Baldwin & Co www.baldwins.co.uk
Just Ingredients www.justingredients.co.uk
Napiers the Herbalist napiers.net/index.html
Naturally Thinking naturallythinking.com
Neal's Yard Remedies www.nealsyardremedies.com

ACKNOWLEDGEMENTS

I would like to thank Liz Woabank for her help in developing my idea for the book and for facilitating that first spine-tingling moment with one of the British Library's original copies of Elizabeth Blackwell's *A Curious Herbal* (1737–39). It's a great honour to be able to share Elizabeth's exquisite illustrations through the publication of this book. To Karin Fremer for her sensitive handling of Elizabeth's illustrations showcasing the beauty of traditional botanical illustration within a setting of clean, contemporary design; and Sally Nicholls for picture research and for scanning the pages on behalf of the British Library. To Alison Moss and the British Library publication team for bringing the book to fruition, with the expert botanical, culinary and editorial advice of Anna Kruger and Becci Woods. To Kim Walker and Vicky Chown of Handmade Apothecary for providing the Foreword, and for their continued support of the book, the herbal community, and the accurate dissemination of the history of medicine. To green-fingered friends, fellow creatives and the Forest Gate Community Garden for ongoing encouragement and much ado about plants, herbs and the botanical world. To Tom for providing me with the many spaces in which to create and evolve such a book, especially our beautiful garden. To Sylvester and Iggy for your love and inspiration, and my family for always being there.

SONYA PATEL ELLIS
is a London-based writer, editor, artist, maker and educator connecting plants and people past, present and future through the prism of A Botanical World, www.abotanicalworld.com. She is also the author of *Collins Botanical Bible/The Botanical Bible* (2018).